Tobacco Control Policy

Strategies, Successes, and Setbacks

Edited by Joy de Beyer and Linda Waverley Brigden

 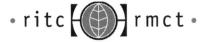

A copublication of the World Bank
and Research for International Tobacco Control (RITC)

Table of Contents

7. Tailoring Tobacco Control Efforts to the Country:
    Prakit Vateesatokit

Figures

Tables

Foreword

Every 10 seconds, someone dies of a tobacco-related disease. This fact is especially painful because the tobacco epidemic is one of the leading preventable causes of death and disability among adults in the world today. In addition, passive smoking has a major effect upon health, especially of children.

Once largely a problem in high-income countries, the epidemic caused by tobacco use has become an enormous and growing problem in many low- and middle-income countries. Already, half of all global deaths from tobacco occur in these countries; by 2025, the proportion will have risen to 70 percent, and the number of tobacco-attributable deaths will exceed 10 million each year. This trend is exacerbated by the efforts of cigarette companies to expand sales in developing countries, where many people are still poorly informed about the harm to health that tobacco causes and many governments have not yet adopted or implemented strong policies to discourage tobacco use.

In one sense, the remedy is simple—not to use tobacco products. But deterring young people from experimenting with cigarettes and encouraging smokers to quit adds up to a big challenge. Most people underestimate the health risks of tobacco use and hugely underestimate how addictive nicotine is and how hard it is to quit. Social norms and pressures to smoke are difficult to counter, especially in the face of aggressive, alluring advertising that associates smoking with success, strength, independence, glamour, and sex. But it can be done, in both developed and developing nations. Advertising and promotion of cigarettes has been and can be stopped. Prices can be raised, and smoking banned in public places. Quit attempts can become more common and more likely to succeed with professional and peer support and help. Tobacco control measures are also extremely cost-effective.

There are many countries where committed individuals, civil society groups, and governments have worked together to define, advocate, legislate, and implement effective tobacco control policies. This book tells the stories of six of these countries, showing how determined and sustained efforts resulted in health-promoting tobacco control policies. These efforts are paying off: the percentage of smokers has declined in many countries, sowing the seeds for long-term gains in health outcomes. There is still much to be done in these six countries and elsewhere around the world. I anticipate that the world's first international health treaty, the Framework Convention on Tobacco Control, will boost national efforts to adopt and implement policies to reduce tobacco use and prevent the unnecessary deaths and disease tobacco causes.

Dr Judith Mackay
Director, Asian Consultancy
on Tobacco Control

Preface

This book was commissioned and published in the hope that descriptions of strategies, successes, and setbacks in promoting stronger tobacco control policies around the world would be of wide interest and might be useful to people grappling with similar issues. As participants in academic, advocacy, and policy meetings on tobacco control, we have been struck by the impact of real-life stories and examples. We have been educated and edified by many excellent presentations and discussions of the principles, practice, and impact of tobacco control policy—but what we remember most clearly, long after, are the stories. We have seen rooms come alive with interest and crackle with energy when people who had been at the center of efforts to develop tobacco control policy related their experiences. So, we decided to record and share some of those stories.

The case studies in this book are addressed to a wide set of readers who share an interest in health issues and policy—people in nongovernmental organizations, community activists, scientists, decisionmakers, health officials, and members of the public. Each story is set in the unique historical, cultural, and political environment of a particular country, but there are common threads and shared lessons that can be applied and adapted in many other countries and circumstances.

Most of the stories are told by advocates, many of them health professionals, who were (and often still are) centrally involved in promoting and developing policies and programs to reduce the harm to health caused by tobacco use. Tobacco control is a contentious issue because strong policies to reduce tobacco use are always opposed by groups with an economic interest in the tobacco industry. This book is not a dispassionate or theoretical analysis of how policies are made but a set of sometimes rather personal accounts and perceptions of how tobacco control policy evolved in six countries and of the strategies, actions, and people that played a role in promoting policies to curb tobacco use. They are stories of commitment, determination, passion, and perseverance—often in the face of formidable opposition. They show how a few committed individuals can bring about change even when confronted with powerful, well-funded opponents. They also document the practical lessons that have been learned in the course of working for policy change.

This book complements (and is quite different from) the numerous scholarly and analytical works on tobacco use and control. The prevalence and health impact of smoking and other forms of tobacco use, within individual countries and globally, have been well documented elsewhere, as has the insidious spread of the epidemic to developing countries.[1] This book does not present data on the negative health impact of tobacco use or estimate the resulting deaths and illnesses, nor is it a political mapping or analysis of the policymaking process. It is, quite literally, a collection of stories about tobacco control policymaking that illustrate the roles that can be played by evidence, advocacy, political and social change, partnerships, media, public relations and public pressure, economic interests, and adversity and opportunity.

The six countries were selected to provide global geographic representation but also because all have made great progress (although to varying degrees) in adopting and implementing sound tobacco control policies. Many other countries also have strategies to share, successes to celebrate, and setbacks to lament—too many to be contained in one volume. In each of the countries represented in this book, there is still much to be done to protect young people and adults from the unnecessary and preventable disease and premature death caused by tobacco use. The narratives gathered here are stories of optimism and of change. It is hoped that they will inspire successful efforts toward developing strong and effective tobacco control policies in other countries.

Joy de Beyer
Linda Waverley Brigden
May 2003

---

1. See, for example, the references cited in chapter 1.

Acknowledgments

The following organizations provided financial support for this book:

- The Human Development Network of the World Bank
- Research for International Tobacco Control (RITC)
- The Office on Smoking and Health of the U.S. Centers for Disease Control and Prevention
- The Tobacco Free Initiative of the World Health Organization.

Special thanks are due to Montasser Kamal who, during his time at RITC, played a key role in commissioning and reviewing the contributions.

We are grateful to the authors who related their countries' stories and to the people who patiently reviewed the drafts and provided additional details and comments or who shared their own papers and archives. In particular, we thank Iraj Abedian, Ed Elmendorf, Vera da Costa e Silva, Yussuf Saloojee, Richard Skolnik, Krisela Steyn, Corné van Walbeek, Nick Wilkins, and Derek Yach.

We also thank copyeditors Ruth Wilson and Yvonne van Ruskenveld of West Coast Editorial Associates and Nancy Levine for the professional polish they brought to the volume.

Contributors

Saifuddin Ahmed is the president of Work for a Better Bangladesh and coordinator of the Bangladesh Anti-Tobacco Alliance. Mr. Ahmed also plays an active role in the SAARC (South Asian Association for Regional Cooperation) Tobacco Control Network and in the Framework Convention Alliance for a strong Framework Convention on Tobacco Control.

Linda Waverley Brigden is the executive director of Research for International Tobacco Control (RITC), an international secretariat housed at Canada's International Development Research Centre (IDRC).

Debra Efroymson is the regional director (Asia) of PATH Canada (Programme for Appropriate Technology in Health, Canada). Ms. Efroymson currently manages tobacco control programs in Bangladesh, India, Nepal, and Vietnam.

Luisa M. da Costa e Silva Goldfarb is the national coordinator of school programs for Brazil's National Tobacco Control Program (NTCP) and has been working in tobacco control since the inception of the NTCP in 1991. From 1999 to 2001, she was a Brazilian delegate on working groups and negotiating bodies for the Framework Convention on Tobacco Control. She has served as executive secretary of the Brazilian inter-ministerial National Commission on Tobacco Use.

Joy de Beyer is an economist who works for the World Bank, coordinating the organization's support for tobacco control around the world.

Ken Kyle heads the Public Issues Office of the Canadian Cancer Society in Ottawa. As a government relations professional, he has played a pivotal role in tobacco control policy issues for more than 15 years.

Rosemary Leaver researched and summarized 4,000 tobacco-related articles that appeared in South African newspapers and magazines over the period 1988–98. The research was conducted as part of the second phase of the Economics of Tobacco Control Project in South Africa at University of Cape Town Applied Fiscal Research Center (AFREC).

Mia Malan is a senior media correspondent in South Africa, covering key health issues. She has received numerous awards for excellence in journalism.

David Sweanor is a lawyer who has worked full time on a wide range of Canadian and global tobacco control issues since 1983. He is the legal counsel to the Non-Smokers' Rights Association and the Smoking and Health Action Foundation, affiliated Canadian nongovernmental organizations.

Prakit Vateesatokit is a professor and dean, Faculty of Medicine, Ramathibodi Hospital, Mahidol University, Bangkok. He is also executive secretary of the Action on Smoking and Health (ASH) Foundation; second vice-chairperson of the Thai Health Promotion Foundation; and a member of the National Committee for the Control of Tobacco Use, Ministry of Public Health.

Witold Zatoński is the director of the Division of Epidemiology and Cancer Prevention at the Maria Sklodowska-Curie Memorial Cancer Centre in Warsaw. His department is the WHO Collaborating Centre on the Action Plan for a Tobacco-Free Europe. He is a member of the Committee of Epidemiology and Public Health at the Polish Academy of Science and has served as a regional coordinator for tobacco control with the International Union against Cancer (UICC).

Abbreviations, Acronyms, and Data Note

ABIFUMO	National Tobacco Manufacturers of Brazil (Associação Brasileira da Indústria de Fumo)
ADHUNIK	Amra Dhumpan Nibaron Kori ("We prevent tobacco") (Bangladesh)
AFTA	ASEAN Free Trade Agreement
AFUBRA	Brazilian Tobacco Growers Association
ANC	African National Congress (South Africa)
ANVISA	National Sanitary Vigilance Agency (Brazil)
APACT	Asia-Pacific Association for the Control of Tobacco
ASEAN	Association of Southeast Asian Nations
ASH	Action on Smoking and Health (successor to TASCP) (Thailand)
BADSA	Body Against Destructive Social Activities (Bangladesh)
BAT	British American Tobacco
BATA	Bangladesh Anti-Tobacco Alliance
BTC	Bangladesh Tobacco Company
CAB	Consumers' Association of Bangladesh
CAT	Coalition Against Tobacco (Bangladesh)
CCCTB	Coordinating Committee for Tobacco Control in Brazil
CCS	Canadian Cancer Society
CCSH	Canadian Council on Smoking and Health
CCSNA	Centre for Clinical Studies on Nicotine Addiction (Brazil)
CDC	Centers for Disease Control and Prevention (United States)
CLACCTA	Latin American Coordinating Committee for Tobacco Control
CONTAPP	National Coordination of Tobacco Control and Primary Cancer Prevention (Brazil)
ETCSA	Economics of Tobacco Control Project in South Africa
EU	European Union

FCTC	Framework Convention on Tobacco Control
FDF	Folk Doctors Foundation (Thailand)
FEDHASA	Federation of Hotel, Liquor and Catering Associations of South Africa
FUNASA	National Health Foundation (Fundação Nacional de Saúde)
GATT	General Agreement on Tariffs and Trade
HSRI	Health Systems Research Institute (Thailand)
IACIB	Institute of Allergy and Clinical Immunology, Bangladesh
IDRC	International Development Research Centre (Canada)
IMF	International Monetary Fund
INB	Intergovernmental Negotiating Body (for the Framework Convention on Tobacco Control)
INCA	National Cancer Institute (Brazil)
LSTB	Law and Society Trust, Bangladesh
MANAS	Madok o Nesha Nirodh Shansthya (Association for the Prevention of Drug Abuse) (Bangladesh)
MANOBIK	Madok Drabya-O-Nesha Birodi Council (Antidrug Council)
MOPH	Ministry of Public Health (Thailand)
NCAS	National Council Against Smoking (South Africa)
NCCTU	National Committee for the Control of Tobacco Use (Thailand)
NCTU	National Commission on Tobacco Use (Brazil)
NGO	nongovernmental organization
NSRA	Non-Smokers' Rights Association (Canada)
NTCP	National Tobacco Control Program (Brazil)
OECD	Organisation for Economic Co-operation and Development
PAHO	Pan American Health Organization
PATH Canada	Programme for Appropriate Technology in Health, Canada
RDA	Rural Doctors' Association (Thailand)
RITC	Research for International Tobacco Control
SAARC	South Asian Association for Regional Cooperation
SABC	South African Broadcasting Corporation
SINDIFUMO	Tobacco Industry Syndicate (Brazil)
TASCP	Thai Anti-Smoking Campaign Project (see ASH)
TAG	Tobacco Action Group (South Africa)
TCCO	Tobacco Consumption Control Office, Ministry of Public Health (Thailand)
TISA	Tobacco Institute of South Africa

TTM	Thai Tobacco Monopoly
UICC	International Union against Cancer
UNICEF	United Nations Children's Fund
USDHHS	U.S. Department of Health and Human Services
WACC	Welfare Association for Cancer Care (Bangladesh)
WBB	Work for a Better Bangladesh
WNTD	World No Tobacco Day
WHO	World Health Organization
YPSA	Young Power in Social Action (Bangladesh)

Data Note

Unless otherwise stated, U.S. dollar amounts are given at the exchange rate prevailing at the time.

1
Overview

Joy de Beyer and Linda Waverley Brigden

Countries around the world are grappling with difficult public health challenges and policy decisions. Disease and death caused by tobacco use, once a problem mainly in high-income countries, have become a large and increasing part of the burden of disease in developing countries.

According to the most recent estimate by the World Health Organization (WHO), 4.9 million people worldwide died in 2000 as a result of their addiction to nicotine, about half of them prematurely (WHO 2002). This huge death toll is rising rapidly, especially in low- and middle-income countries, where most of the world's 1.2 billion tobacco users live. As shown in figure 1.1, developing countries already account for half of all deaths attributable to tobacco. The proportion will rise to 7 out of 10 by 2025 because smoking prevalence has been increasing in many low- and middle-income countries even as it is falling in richer countries, especially among men. Developing countries also account for about half of the world disease burden related to tobacco (figure 1.2). And tobacco use has far-reaching indirect effects on human health and the economy, in addition to the direct harm it causes.[1]

But the course and pattern of this epidemic can be changed. The policies that are effective in encouraging tobacco users to quit and dissuading young people from starting are well known and proven. Many countries have managed to change behavior, reduce the prevalence of tobacco use, and ease the burden of tobacco-related disease and death. This book describes recent struggles, successes, and setbacks in six countries on six continents, where the efforts of public health practitioners, researchers, activists, policymakers, politicians, and the press have achieved sound tobacco control policies even in the face of enormous opposition from those who profit from these deadly products.

Reducing the devastating health damage caused by tobacco use is especially difficult because of nicotine's powerful addictive properties,

---

1. For studies on the prevalence of tobacco use and on the associated health and economic effects, see, for example, Murray and Lopez (1996); WHO (1997); World Bank (1999); Corrao and others (2000); Jha and Chaloupka (2000); and Mackay and Eriksen (2002).

Figure 1.1. Deaths Attributable to Selected Leading Risk Factors, Worldwide, 2000

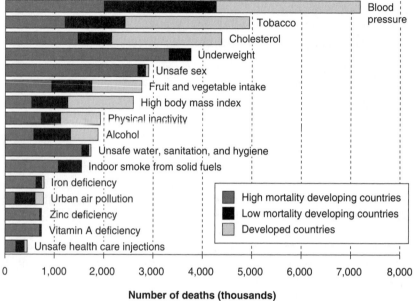

Source: WHO 2002.

low prices for tobacco products, well-established social norms, and constant inducements to smoke, fueled by billions of dollars worth of tobacco industry advertising and promotion. Low prices and advertising can be countered by policies that raise taxes on tobacco products and outlaw all advertising and promotion of these products. Such policies are likely to have an even stronger effect in reducing tobacco use if complemented by good public information on the associated health risks (for instance, through strong, large warnings on cigarette packs), by bans on smoking in public spaces, and by advice and help to people who want to quit.

Why These Six Countries?

The six countries whose stories are told in this book—Bangladesh, Brazil, Canada, Poland, South Africa, and Thailand—are at very different stages of development and of the tobacco epidemic (see table 1.1). Brazil and Bangladesh are two to six times more populous than any of the other four countries. With regard to wealth and social indicators such as child malnutrition and illiteracy rates, Canada, a developed country, is at one extreme and Bangladesh at the other. Life expectancy at birth is consider-

Figure 1.2. Disease Burden Attributable to Selected Leading Risk Factors, Worldwide, 2000

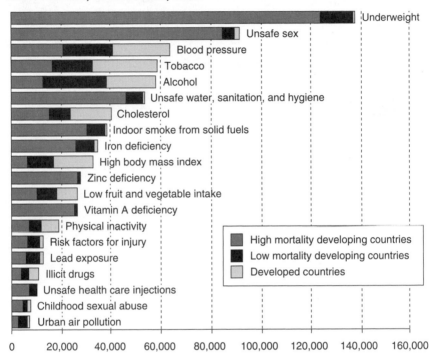

Number of disability-adjusted life years (thousands)

Source: WHO 2002.

ably higher in Canada than in any of the other countries; it is lowest in South Africa, as a result of the ravages of AIDS.

The six countries also differ in the strength and history of their tobacco control policies and in the extent to which they are succeeding in reducing tobacco use. The share of adult men who regularly use tobacco is around 40 percent in five of the countries. In Canada it is substantially lower, 27 percent, down from a peak of 60 percent in 1960 (Smoking and Health Action Foundation 2000). Male smoking prevalence has fallen significantly in three of the other countries: in South Africa, from well over 50 percent in the early 1990s to 42 percent in 1998 (Corrao and others 2000; van Walbeek 2002); in Thailand, from 49 percent in 1986 to 38 percent in 1999 (Vateesatokit et al 2000); and in the most dramatic case, that of Poland, from peak levels of 65–75 percent in the mid-1970s to 39 percent in 1998 (Corrao and others 2000). It is no coincidence that, as table 1.1 shows, compared to the other middle- and high-income countries, cigarettes are (relatively) the

Table 1.1. Indicators of Development, Tobacco Use, Health Impact, and Cigarette Prices in Six Countries

Indicator	Bangladesh	Brazil	Canada	Poland	South Africa	Thailand
General						
GDP per capita, 2001 (U.S. dollars)	370	3,060	21,340	4,240	2,900	1,970
Population, 2001 (millions)	133.4	172.5	31.0	38.6	43.2	61.2
Life expectancy at birth, 2000	61	68	79	73	48	69
Percentage of children under 5 malnourished[a]	48	6	0	0	9	19
Illiteracy (percent)						
Adult women	69	14	0	0	15	6
Adult men	47	15	0	0	14	3
Tobacco use by adults						
Percentage of adults who are regular users[b]						
Men	40	38	27	39	42	38
Women[c]	10–(50?)	29	23	19	11	2
Per capita annual cigarette consumption[d]	245	1,802	1,976	3,291	1,516	1,067
Health impact						
Lung cancer rate per 100,000 population[e]						
Male	79	45	79	162/510	100	21
Female	12	14	34/77	43	24	7

Table 1.1. continued

Indicator	Bangladesh	Brazil	Canada	Poland	South Africa	Thailand
Lip, mouth, and pharynx cancer rate per 100,000 population						
Male	65	15	9	19/26	47	3
Female	49	3	3/6	4	9	2
Cigarette prices, March 2001						
Local brand (U.S. dollars)	0.83	0.80	2.88	1.13	1.34	0.69
Imported brand (U.S. dollars)	1.26	0.85	3.40	1.51	1.34	1.26
Minutes of labor to buy pack of local brand of cigarettes	106	17–18[f]	16–17[g]	40	20	23
Minutes of labor to buy 1 kilogram of rice	76–89[h]	11–13	9–11	23	9	14
Minutes of labor to buy a Big Mac hamburger	435[i]	36–45	13–14	54	19	43

a. Less than 2 standard deviations below international reference median weight for age.

b. For Bangladesh, Poland, and South Africa, data are for 1998; for Brazil, 1995; for Canada and Thailand, 1999.

c. About 10 percent of adult Bangladeshi women smoke cigarettes, but many more chew tobacco. There is no national statistic on chewing prevalence, but one nongovernmental organization, Naripokho, estimates it at about 50 percent among adult women, which would be similar to India's rate.

d. For Bangladesh, Canada, Poland, and Thailand, data are for 1995; for Brazil, 1990; for South Africa, 1997.

e. Cancers of trachea, lung, and bronchus. Data are for adults age 35 and older (Brazil and Thailand) or 45 and older (Bangladesh and South Africa), and 45–64/65 and older (Poland). For Canada, oral cancers include cancers of the tongue, gum, mouth, and pharynx, and are for all ages, 1999. Lung cancer data for Canada are also for all ages.

f. Data are for Rio de Janeiro and São Paulo.

g. Data are for Montreal and Toronto.

h. Range is 76 for coarse rice, 89 for medium rice.

i. Big Macs are not sold in Bangladesh; this is for a comparable "Wimpy" Hamburger.

Source: World Bank 2002; Corrao and others 2000; Guindon, Tobin, and Yach 2002; Health Canada; Cancer Institute and Center (Warsaw); Bangladesh Bureau of Statistics.

least affordable in Poland, where a person earning the average wage must work for about 40 minutes to earn the price of a pack of cigarettes—roughly twice as long as in the other four countries in the same or high income category (Guindon, Tobin, and Yach 2002). In Bangladesh, very low wage rates make cigarettes least affordable of all the countries, even though the prices (of local brands) are among the lowest.

This is a very heterogeneous group of countries. But there is a common thread: all six have achieved notable successes in tobacco control policymaking by building advocacy on sound research and evidence. Their stories exemplify important features of policymaking, particularly the significant role that can be played by determined individuals and by civil society groups.

The stories make it clear that there is no magic formula. Instead, they tell of policy entrepreneurs (Kingdon 1995)—both individuals and groups—willing to champion the issue; of politicians committed to public health and to placing tobacco control on the policy agenda; of researchers who have published and publicized compelling national or international data; and of national, regional, and international political, social, economic, and policy environments that supported action on this important issue.

Many other countries, or states and provinces within countries, have achieved admirable successes in tobacco control policymaking and could have been included in this book, were it not for the limitations of space. We hope that the inspiring experiences of other countries will be related elsewhere.

Each country included in this book has some extraordinary accomplishments in tobacco control policy and its own particular strengths. In Bangladesh systematic, concerted, and methodical efforts by nongovernmental organizations (NGOs) provide a model of very low-budget but effective advocacy against what seemed to be impossible odds. In Brazil, by contrast, persistent action led from within the government resulted in strong legislation and a nationwide, decentralized program, with training and support cascading down the levels of government.

Canada has long been a world leader in tobacco control legislation, taxation, and health warnings, backed by strong citizen and political support. It provides a model of coalition building among civil society groups that resulted in well-planned, systematic advocacy initiatives.

In Poland and South Africa dramatic political and social change created new environments and policy windows that public health advocates were able to turn to their advantage. In the 1990s these countries enacted, relatively quickly, strong, comprehensive legislation—in both cases, in two legislative steps, with a second law strengthening the first. Both countries began with policies to better inform consumers and to restrict smoking and advertising. At a later stage, tax increases were put in place and helped reduce consumption. Each country had strong, charismatic champions who helped drive the issue, through undaunted, persistent efforts over many years. And in both countries the availability of strong local research evidence, especially on the economic implications of tax increases, was enormously important.

In Thailand, as in Bangladesh, an NGO played a pivotal role. Tobacco control policy has been significantly influenced by strong advocates in the health sector with direct access to government officials, some of whom showed great political courage, integrity, and commitment to serving the best interests of the Thai people.

Although all of the stories describe setbacks and disappointments, none of them dwells on mistakes made or opportunities missed, or on what could have been done better. There are lessons to be learned from both the successes and the setbacks in each country. The stories describe how advocates and policymakers changed their strategies in certain countries as they learned from their mistakes and built on their achievements.

What Factors Made the Difference?

Although each country's situation and story is unique, there are commonalities across the six countries—lessons and experiences that are also applicable in other contexts.

- In each case, legislative successes were won in the face of vigorous opposition from a tobacco industry striving to defend its profits and market. Sometimes the legislation was weakened or delayed or its implementation was inhibited. Compromises had to be made, but these sometimes paved the way for stronger follow-up laws a few years later.
- Time and again, a key role was played by NGOs and by individuals— often very charismatic people—who showed extraordinary commitment and dedication. Through their knowledge and perseverance, they became credible spokespersons for their cause and won the ear of policymakers.
- Coalitions of individuals and organizations brought new skills and perspectives to bear on the issue. Broad-based groups such as consumers' rights groups, development agencies, women's rights activists, lawyers, and religious organizations made important contributions. Personal and institutional objectives and prestige were sometimes set aside for the sake of achieving common goals. Groups had to grapple with the organizational and relationship issues that are part of maintaining a smoothly functioning coalition. Not all coalitions survived.

- Effective advocacy has to be learned. Tobacco control advocates found that change is a slow, evolutionary process; they learned to expect setbacks and make use of them to turn defeats into victories; to take advantage of favorable opportunities as they arose, developing rapid-response, short-term strategies as well as long-term goals; and to be creative in seeking allies. Not least, they learned about the need for optimism and for a continuous, sustained effort.
- While much can be done with little money if funds are used wisely, lack of an organizational home and a minimal level of financial resources can make it hard to operate effectively. Working collaboratively with national and international agencies can help provide access to sustained, if limited, resources.
- Strong political support and political champions are absolutely crucial to success. At times, political champions have had to persuade and win over (or prevail over) their own colleagues. Public opinion polls have been influential in some countries, demonstrating to politicians clear popular support for strong policies to protect children and adults from the harm caused by tobacco use.
- Amazing transformations in social norms can occur, spurred by changes in legislation, shifts in the socioeconomic context, and better public information. This is starkly evident to anyone who choked through meetings in smoke-filled rooms in Poland in the late 1980s and has had the pleasure of visiting Poland again in recent years and enjoying smoke-free meetings and meals. The media can have a powerful effect in influencing popular opinion and paving the way for legislation. Legislation both reflects and reinforces—or institutionalizes—changing social norms.
- An understanding of the political framework and the legislative timetable of the country contributes to effective advocacy. That understanding might involve knowing when to intervene and whom to target; cultivating legislators who are favorably disposed to an issue; or recognizing when an idea's time has come and responding swiftly with information and advocacy.
- Legislation must be coupled with strong attention to implementation and enforcement. This can be an even greater challenge than getting the legislation through with its teeth intact. Often, legislation is only a first step, and regulations or further actions are required before provisions can be implemented and take effect.
- Sound research and evidence are extremely important as a basis for good policy decisions. Evidence and research findings from other countries can be compelling, but there is also likely to be a need for strategic, selective local studies and data, presented concisely and graphically. Building, publishing, and widely publicizing a solid infor-

mation base proved enormously useful to policymakers and advocates and helped promote changes in public attitudes and awareness that gradually led to changes in social norms in several countries.

- Tobacco control policies and strategies must be comprehensive. It is now well recognized that single initiatives are not enough; real impact comes from a combination of education and information, legislation, taxation, community action, professional involvement, prevention and cessation programs in various settings, prohibitions on smoking in public places, and complete bans on advertising and promotion of tobacco and tobacco brands.

- Strong, effective tobacco control policy that includes tax increases and complementary health promotion efforts relies on success in bringing together diverse interest groups and finding common ground. This is especially important with regard to the ministries of health and finance, whose objectives of sound fiscal management and better public health outcomes can both be furthered by tobacco tax increases.

- Not all policymakers were won over by data on tobacco-related morbidity and mortality. In Bangladesh reframing the issue to focus on the contribution of tobacco use to malnutrition was what captured the attention of policymakers. Donor agencies may be more interested in and willing to support tobacco control to the extent that it contributes to and relates to broader development issues.

- Not long ago, in some countries, the situation seemed hopeless. Efforts by poorly funded public health groups were opposed by tobacco companies with powerful political connections and deep pockets. Social norms favored smoking, and many people were skeptical about or even hostile to tobacco control efforts. But, as in Canada, public health proponents discovered that "seemingly irresistible forces within the tobacco industry could be successfully challenged by effective advocacy" (Sweanor and Kyle, ch. 4 in this volume).

- Persistence is essential. Never give up.

The Big Picture

Each country profiled in this book has recorded great progress and substantial achievements in tobacco control policy. But in none of them is victory assured, and in none has the war against misinformation, ignorance, addiction, preventable disease, and premature death been won. Smoking still claims too many lives, and too many teenagers are enticed into trying "just one" and then another, starting what will become a deadly addiction that most will regret ever taking up and will later struggle to break.

This is an important time—perhaps a watershed—in the history of tobacco control policy and of efforts to curb the epidemic caused by tobacco use. The negotiations for an international Framework Convention on Tobacco Control (FCTC) have provided an important forum and process, enabling each of the 165 participating countries to weigh competing national interests carefully and decide how strongly committed they are to measures that can improve health outcomes by reducing tobacco use. The challenge that lies ahead for countries is to ratify the FCTC and to strengthen national legislation, policies, and programs and international cooperation to reduce tobacco use.

Sometimes the discussion about tobacco control is framed as health versus economics, with people conceding the harm that tobacco does to health but emphasizing the economic contributions of the tobacco industry in the form of jobs, incomes, exports, and tax revenues. The relative economic importance of the tobacco industry, however, is often exaggerated, and the economic costs of tobacco should also be considered. These costs include the direct and indirect costs of medical care; the loss of productivity and earnings as a result of tobacco-related illnesses and deaths; environmental degradation caused by pesticides and the use of firewood for curing tobacco; and fires caused by lit cigarettes and matches.

Perhaps most insidious is the harm done to poor smokers and their families by the diversion of scarce family income to buy tobacco products. The chapter on Bangladesh presents detailed data on the opportunity cost of tobacco purchases, comparing the cost of cigarettes with the costs of food staples that the money spent on cigarettes might have bought—this in a country where perhaps half of all adults smoke or chew tobacco while nearly half of all children under five are malnourished. As Efroymson and others (2001) have shown, "Each tobacco user represents one or more people—whether the smoker or his or her spouse or child—who is needlessly going hungry." Although this situation is not well documented in many other countries, it is certainly not unique to Bangladesh; for example, women in a poor village in Sri Lanka said that cigarettes were the leading cause of poverty in their village (Skolnik 2003). National surveys of household expenditure find that in Egypt and India 2 to 3 percent of all household expenditures go for tobacco products; in South Africa, families that include at least one smoker and that are in the lowest income quartile spent 4.7 percent of their income on cigarettes in 1995 (Basheer 1993; van Walbeek 2000; Sayginsoy 2002). For families living on the edge of poverty, even small amounts can make an enormous difference to family well-being.

It is thus misleading to frame the tobacco control debate as "health versus economics." Tobacco generates income for some but entails large costs for others. Tobacco control is clearly key to promoting health and preventing unnecessary deaths, and it can be achieved in the context of sound economic and social policies, without harming economies. Brazil's discussions with tobacco farmers and its initiatives to work with them are a case in point.

Tobacco is clearly much more than a health issue; it has significant economic implications and can have an impact on economic development. Improvements in health can contribute to sustained and substantial improvements in social and economic well-being, as the WHO Commission on Macroeconomics and Health (2001) recently emphasized. Conversely, poor health can undermine social and economic development. The broader development issues relating to tobacco and its control have been much discussed in the FCTC deliberations. The FCTC has the potential to provide a common framework allowing countries to move ahead together to reduce tobacco use, mindful both of those—particularly among the poor—who will benefit and of those whose livelihoods may be jeopardized if national and global markets for tobacco decline.

Global partnerships, both explicit and implicit, can work to the common good of citizens in all countries. There is great value in comparing notes with other countries, learning from their successes and mistakes, and borrowing their data. Governments often hesitate to step out ahead of the pack but can be emboldened by the actions of others, as shown by the domino effect of changes in tax policy, advertising bans, and the recently introduced large pictorial health warnings on cigarette packs.

We hope that this book will help inspire and inform tobacco control activists, public health practitioners, policymakers, and citizens who care about their health and the futures of their children, so that more can be done to reduce the harm that tobacco does to health and lives around the world.

References

Bangladesh Bureau of Statistics. 2000. *Statistical Yearbook of Baugladesh, 2000.* Dhaka, Bangladesh.

Basheer, R. A. 1993. "The Economics of Tobacco and Its Consumption in India." Report prepared for the World Bank. Washington, D.C. Processed.

Commission on Macroeconomics and Health. 2001. "Macroeconomics and Health: Investing in Health for Economic Development." World Health Organization, Geneva.

Corrao, M. A., G. E. Guindon, N. Sharma, and D. F. Shokoohi, eds. 2000. "Tobacco Control Country Profiles." American Cancer Society, Atlanta, Ga.

Efroymson, D., S. Ahmed, J. Townsend, S. Alam, A. Dey, R. Shah, B. Dhar, A. Sujon, K. Ahmed, and O. Rahman. 2001. "Hungry for Tobacco: An Analysis of the Economic Impact of Tobacco Consumption on the Poor in Bangladesh." *Tobacco Control* 10 (3): 212–17. Available at <http://tc.bmjjournals.com/cgi/content/full/10/3/212>.

Guindon, G. E., S. Tobin, and D. Yach. 2002. "Trends and Affordability of Cigarette Prices: Ample Room for Tax Increases and Related Health Gains." *Tobacco Control* 11 (1): 35–43. Available at <http://tc.bmjjournals.com/cgi/content/full/11/1/35>.

Health Canada. Cancer Surveillance On-Line. Available at <http://cythera.ic.gc.ca/dsol/cancer/help_e.html>.

Jha, P., and F. J. Chaloupka, eds. 2000. *Tobacco Control in Developing Countries.* New York: Oxford University Press for the World Bank and the World Health Organization.

Kingdon, J. W. 1995. *Agendas, Alternatives, and Public Policies.* 2d ed. New York: HarperCollins College Publishers.

Mackay, J., and M. Eriksen. 2002. *The Tobacco Atlas.* Geneva: World Health Organization.

Murray, C. J., and A. D. Lopez, eds. 1996. *The Global Burden of Disease: A Comprehensive Assessment of Mortality and Disability from Diseases, Injuries and Risk Factors in 1990 and Projected to 2020.* Cambridge, Mass.: Harvard School of Public Health.

Sayginsoy, Ö. 2002. "An Analysis of the Links between Poverty and Tobacco in Egypt." World Bank, Washington, D.C. Processed.

Skolnik, R. 2003. Personal communication.

Smoking and Health Action Foundation, Canada. 2000. "Framework Convention on Tobacco Control. An International Instrument to Deal with an International Problem." Submission to the World Health Organization. Available at Non-Smokers' Rights Association Website, <http://www.nsra-adnf.ca/english/FCTC%20brief%20(SHAF)%20August%202000.html>; accessed February 25, 2003.

van Walbeek, C. P. 2000. "The Distributional Impact of Changes in Tobacco Prices: Some Preliminary Findings." Economics of Tobacco Control Project (Phase II). University of Cape Town, South Africa. Processed.

———. 2002. "The Economics of Tobacco Control in South Africa." University of Cape Town, South Africa.

Vateesatokit, P., B. Hughes, and B. Ritthphakdee. 2000. "Thailand: Winning Battles, but the War's Far from Over." *Tobacco Control* 9(2):122–7. Available at <http://tc.bmjjournals.com/cgi/content/full/9/2/122>.

WHO (World Health Organization). 1997. "Tobacco or Health: A Global Status Report." Geneva.

———. 2002. *The World Health Report 2002: Reducing Risks, Promoting Healthy Life.* Geneva.

World Bank. 1999. *Curbing the Epidemic: Governments and the Economics of Tobacco Control.* Development in Practice series. Washington, D.C.

———. 2002. *World Development Indicators 2002.* Washington, D.C. Selected portions of the database are available at <http://www.worldbank.org/data/wdi2002/index.htm>.

2

Building Momentum
for Tobacco Control:
The Case of Bangladesh

Debra Efroymson and Saifuddin Ahmed

Bangladesh is a small, poor, densely populated country of roughly 130 million people, about 80 percent of whom live in rural areas. It has a well-deserved reputation as being disaster-prone, having been stricken with droughts, floods, and a range of health and environmental problems, from dengue and cholera to arsenic contamination of the water supply. It should come as no surprise, then, that tobacco control has not gained much attention or been considered a priority. With so many competing causes of disease, and with nearly half the population living below the poverty line and consuming less than 2,122 calories per day (Bangladesh Bureau of Statistics 1998a), tobacco has generally seemed too remote and insignificant an issue to be on the country's agenda of concerns. Yet tobacco use is widespread and increasing rapidly, and knowledge about the harm it causes to health is slight. Moreover, although other causes of death still dominate, tobacco use contributes a nontrivial amount to the overall burden of disease and death. And it has clear and significant immediate negative effects on the welfare of poor families, when scarce resources that could be used for food are instead spent on tobacco.

From the late 1980s through most of the 1990s, tobacco control remained the domain of a few groups: Amra Dhumpan Nibaron Kori (ADHUNIK), which, roughly translated, means, "We prevent tobacco"; the Bangladesh Cancer Society; Madok o Nesha Nirodh Shansthya (MANAS—the Association for the Prevention of Drug Abuse); and the National Non-Smokers' Forum. Although these groups achieved some significant successes, for the most part tobacco control remained a fringe activity that received wide publicity on World No Tobacco Day, May 31, and was then forgotten for the rest of the year.

But in 1999 the tide began to turn. The aggressive activities of British American Tobacco (BAT) pushed the advocates toward stronger action. For the first time, a number of organizations got together and coordinated their activities. A coalition emerged, a High Court victory was obtained, and tobacco control in Bangladesh finally began to assume some of the importance and receive some of the attention it had long warranted. By late 2002, strong new legislation had been submitted for consideration by Parliament.

This case study discusses the dynamic process of tobacco control policymaking in one developing country and the role that advocates can play in informing and influencing the process. The ultimate goal has not yet been reached, but the journey has begun.

Tobacco in the Lives of the Bangladeshi People

Although Bangladesh is a Muslim country and tobacco is generally considered *haram* (forbidden) under Islam, tobacco use is widespread. The Bangladesh Bureau of Statistics regularly conducts surveys that monitor, among other things, smoking rates. As table 2.1 shows, smoking rates are higher among men than women. In 1997 the highest reported rate (70.3 percent) was for men age 35–49, while the lowest (0.1 percent) was for girls age 10–14.

A significant flaw in the prevalence measures is that they cover only smoking, not tobacco consumption as a whole. Tobacco chewing is common in Bangladesh, particularly among women. A study by Naripokho, a nongovernmental organization (NGO) working on women's issues, indicates that the rate for use of all forms of tobacco, smokeless and smoked, by women is around 50 percent, but no nationwide or large-scale surveys exist to verify this finding (Haq 2001).

According to data compiled by the World Health Organization (WHO) on tobacco and cigarette production and consumption in Bangladesh, an estimated 70 percent of the tobacco produced is used for cigarettes and *bidis* (small cigarettes handrolled in paper), 20 percent is consumed as chewing tobacco, and the remainder is used in cigars, snuff, and pipe tobacco. In 1997, 16,500 million cigarettes were manufactured, consisting

Table 2.1. Smoking Rates by Age and Sex, Bangladesh, 1997 (percent)

Sex	Age				
---	10–14	15–19	20–34	35–49	50+
Male	2.8	14.4	47.6	70.3	21.2
Female	0.1	0.9	3.3	6.6	2.8
Average for both sexes	1.6	8.3	23.7	41.0	12.3

Source: Bangladesh Bureau of Statistics (1999).

of 2,900 million filter and 13,600 million nonfilter cigarettes. Since the mid-1980s, Bangladesh has had a growing negative trade balance in tobacco and tobacco products as leaf imports have increased strongly (see table 2.2). In 1993 export earnings amounted to US$10 million, half of the US$20 million that was spent on tobacco and tobacco product imports. By 1995, according to the World Bank, the negative net earnings from tobacco trade (leaves and cigarettes) had nearly tripled, to US$27.8 million.

Although tobacco is available in a multitude of forms in Bangladesh, only cigarette packages carry a warning. This states (in Bengali), in small type, "Government warning: smoking is deleterious to health." The same warning is used on BAT billboards and on television advertisements but not on advertisements for cigarettes produced by other companies or for bidis. What little information is conveyed in the warning is inaccessible to

Table 2.2. Annual Tobacco Trade and Agricultural Statistics, Bangladesh, Selected Years, 1970–98

Indicator	1970	1980	1990	1995	1998
Cigarette imports (millions of sticks)	—	177	86	70	52
Cigarette exports (millions of sticks)	—	—	2	—	47
Tobacco leaf imports (metric tons)	—	740	805	1,137	5,012
Tobacco leaf exports					
Metric tons	—	—	870	278	2,307
Percentage of total exports	—	—	0.11	0.02	—
Cigarette production (millions of sticks)	17,787	13,830	12,289	17,379	—
Tobacco leaf production (metric tons)	41,200	39,524	37,800	38,000	36,655
Land devoted to growing tobacco					
Hectares	45,700	45,091	45,070	36,000	32,823
Percentage of agricultural land	0.50	0.49	0.48	0.44	—
Employment in tobacco manufacturing (number of workers)	4,190	6,340	27,155	—	—

— Not available.
Source: Corrao and others 2000.

the large proportion of the population unable to read. According to the Bangladesh Bureau of Statistics (1999), in 1997 only 42 percent of females and 51 percent of males over age 7 were literate.

The law has yet to set a standard for informing tobacco users about the range of diseases caused by smoking and tobacco use. One study found that while more than 93 percent of male smokers and more than 84 percent of female smokers know that smoking is generally bad for health, far fewer are aware of specific effects such as cancer, respiratory diseases, stroke, and heart disease. In general, nonsmokers have slightly higher awareness of the diseases caused by smoking than do smokers (Bangladesh Bureau of Statistics 1996).

Although the lack of nationwide statistics on tobacco use makes tracking the epidemic difficult, a few facts are clear. Tobacco use (as distinguished from smoking) is widespread among men and women. Most users are not aware of the health effects, and written warnings can be read by only about half the population. Better statistics are needed to track tobacco use among the population and to monitor changes when tobacco control laws and interventions come into effect.

The Tobacco Industry in Bangladesh

The Bangladesh Tobacco Company (BTC) operated essentially as a monopoly for many years. It was originally a subsidiary of BAT, which has been doing business in Bangladesh since 1954. In the late 1990s BAT bought controlling shares in the BTC, which then began operating directly as BAT.

BAT reported pretax profits in 1998 of US$15.4 million and had a budget of US$3.34 million for brand promotion and development (BAT 1998). This huge promotion budget explains the ubiquitous presence of BAT brands (mostly Benson & Hedges and John Player Gold Leaf and, to a lesser extent, 555) on billboards, in newspaper advertisements, and in cigarette display cases, as well as in television advertisements and at concerts sponsored by Benson & Hedges. BAT advertises its cheaper brand, Star, less widely, mostly on inexpensive posters on the street.

About 15 local companies also produce cigarettes, which are less expensive than BAT's. The largest manufacturer of bidis is Akiz Bidi, which also produces the Navy brand. Various cheaper brands are advertised to some extent through posters, on small signs in shops, and in display cases, but Navy is the only non-BAT brand for which there is any extensive advertising.

Researchers monitored the advertisements on ATN Bangla (a Bengali-language Indian satellite television station) from 8 p.m. to 10 p.m. on a Saturday evening, a time when young people are fairly likely to be watching television (Shaha, Dhar, and Efroymson 2000). During the two-hour period, they counted 38 tobacco advertisements, covering 14 minutes and 13 seconds. There were advertisements for two different brands of bidis and seven different brands of cigarettes. Ten advertisements for Navy brand ran during the two hours. Many of the advertisements conveyed the message that smoking makes one strong, healthy, and irresistible to women. Two examples illustrate the point:

- An oxcart gets stuck in the mud, and the driver is unable to push it out. A young man approaches, watched with great admiration by a pretty peasant girl. He takes a few puffs of a cigarette, then pushes the oxcart out of the mud and offers a cigarette to the driver. The girl is in ecstasy.
- Mr. Navy rescues a young woman from drowning. She turns out to have been faking the incident, but she wins his affection by calling him back to retrieve the pack of Navy cigarettes that fell from his pocket while he tried to resuscitate her. They frolic on the beach, then stand lovingly while he smokes.

These advertisements carry a health warning in Bengali, but it is flashed briefly either at the beginning or the end of the ad, so quickly and in such small type that it is virtually impossible to read, even by the half of the population that is literate. In any case, it simply repeats the statutory warning that is printed on cigarette packs: "Smoking is deleterious to health." The High Court of Bangladesh, in response to a petition brought by members of the Bangladesh Anti-Tobacco Alliance (BATA), recently held that this mode of flashing the warning is in violation of the law. The court went on to say that all tobacco advertising should be banned. The case is currently on appeal.

As part of its attempt to resist regulation, BAT has promoted itself as a responsible company. It has done this in several ways:

- In 2001 the company issued a voluntary code of conduct that limited tobacco advertisements on television and radio to the hours of 10 p.m. to 6 a.m. (BAT 2000).
- BAT claims that it offers samples only to smokers or tobacco users over 18 years of age.
- In newspaper advertisements and in programs distributed at cultural events sponsored by BAT, messages such as "Our events promote more than just our brands" are displayed.
- A tree nursery program supported by BAT has brought the company much positive attention. The minister of the environment has visited the Dhaka nursery, and the trees and accompanying advertising signs line some medians in Chittagong, the main port city. In August 2001

BAT set up highly publicized roadside stands in Dhaka to hand out tree saplings.

- On July 28, 2001, BAT launched a so-called Youth Smoking Prevention Campaign consisting of 30-second television advertisements, three 1-minute radio scripts, billboards, and stickers. In all the materials, BAT claimed that smoking is an adult choice, that those under age 18 should not smoke, and that BAT feels a responsibility to curtail and prevent youth smoking. More astute young people easily see through this campaign and recognize the contradiction between the company's heavily advertising its brands and yet telling youths not to smoke (WBB and PATH Canada 2001). For many, however, the campaign seems to offer evidence of how responsible and well-meaning BAT is, and it provides a further excuse for the inaction of lawmakers who wish to avoid passing tough laws to control tobacco.

The Economics of Tobacco in Bangladesh

The government of Bangladesh has sent mixed messages about tobacco. Former prime minister Sheikh Hasina has said that tobacco spending is a waste of money and that redirecting the money spent toward food purchases could lower the rate of malnutrition (BATA 2001). Yet Hasina's government awarded BAT a trophy for being one of the country's largest exporters. BAT is apparently the biggest taxpayer in the country, with reported tax payments in 1998 of approximately US$5.55 million (BAT 1998).

But export earnings and tax payments do not provide a complete economic picture of the tobacco industry in Bangladesh. Missing are such items as the trade deficit, the costs associated with tobacco-related health problems, and the effect of smokers purchasing tobacco rather than food. In fiscal year 1997–98 Bangladesh earned US$5.4 million in tobacco exports, but it also imported US$19.93 million worth of tobacco, for a net loss of over US$14.4 million (Bangladesh Bureau of Statistics 1998b). Although figures on health costs associated with tobacco use are not available, the Bangladesh Cancer Society estimates that half of the annual deaths from cancer in Bangladesh (75,000 people) result from tobacco use.

The tobacco industry also has an effect on employment. Cigarettes require very little labor to manufacture. Bidi rolling is much more labor-intensive, but most of the profits are absorbed by middlemen, with the laborers, almost exclusively women and children, earning a pittance for their many hours of grueling work in uncomfortable and unhealthy settings (UNICEF 2000). According to the World Bank (1999), because most goods and services in Bangladesh require a larger labor input than cigarettes, a shift from tobacco product use and manufacturing to other products and services could mean a tremendous boon for employment.

Although tobacco is perceived as being cheap, its actual cost, compared with food, education, and health care, is quite high—exorbitantly so for those for whom basic survival is a daily struggle. A study on tobacco and poverty (Efroymson and others 2001) revealed that tobacco is most commonly used by those who can least afford it. The smoking rate among the poorest (those with a household income of less than US$20 per month) is 58.2 percent, while for the wealthiest (those with a household income of more than US$100 per month), it is 32.3 percent. On average across the country, spending for tobacco represents 2.8 percent of total income, from a low of 1.5 percent for households with total spending of less than US$18 per month to a high of 4.4 percent for households spending more than US$472 per month. The amount spent by the average male cigarette smoker in 1997 would purchase 2,942 calories of rice per day—enough to make a difference between family members getting by or suffering from malnutrition.

Between 1992 and 1996, annual per capita cigarette consumption increased by 33 percent, from 100 to 133 sticks. Meanwhile annual per capita egg consumption fell by 29 percent, from 17 to 12 eggs. In other words, per capita consumption in 1996 was 1 egg and 11 cigarettes per month. Average per capita expenditure on tobacco is almost half per capita expenditure for health, and more than half the amount spent on education. In both urban and rural areas, per capita expenditure is higher for tobacco than for milk. At 2000 prices, the money needed to purchase one pack of BAT's John Player Gold Leaf regular cigarettes would buy more than a dozen eggs, or more than a kilogram of lentils, or more than a liter of soybean oil, or half a kilogram of beef. BAT Bangladesh's gross turnover in cigarettes for 1998 (US$293 million) could have purchased 4.7 billion eggs, or enough to feed almost 13 million children one egg per day (Efroymson and others 2001).

Efroymson and others (2001) estimate that 10.5 million children who are currently going hungry would have enough to eat if their parents redirected 69 percent of their tobacco expenditures to food. Malnutrition wreaks havoc on the Bangladesh economy: UNICEF (1998) estimates that lost lives, disability, and productivity losses caused by malnutrition cost Bangladesh the equivalent of more than 5 percent of its gross national product.

So far, research and publicity have not sufficiently impressed on policymakers and the public the negative economic impact of tobacco use in Bangladesh. As long as BAT is able to convince policymakers that the company is a positive factor in the economy, advocates are unlikely to succeed in obtaining strong tobacco control laws and policies.

Whatever the features peculiar to Bangladesh, in many ways the tobacco situation is like that in many other countries, particularly those with a similar economic status. The tobacco industry, as in most countries, is dominated by a transnational company; tobacco use is widespread, as is ignorance of the effects of its use; and policymakers and civil society have a distance to travel to recognize the harm that tobacco does and to be convinced of the need for tobacco control legislation.

A Chronicle of Tobacco Control in Bangladesh

Until recently, tobacco control advocacy and activities were limited, and hopes and aspirations concerning the issue were generally modest. This was partly because of the many health problems that face Bangladesh but perhaps also because public health advocates felt overwhelmed and discouraged in the face of BAT's enormous influence, resources, and visibility. Then the industry went too far and sparked an extraordinary reaction, the outcome of which has given new hope and a new impetus to tobacco control efforts.

In the following necessarily simplified account, the key role played by various NGOs in studying the problem, promoting solutions, and influencing key players is evident. The government and the judicial system have also played a critical part, as have the media and the general public.

Early Concern about Tobacco Use

Although the issue of tobacco use has always attracted some interest in Bangladesh, it has mainly been perceived as a problem only by people concerned about cancer and drug use. Tobacco control was taken on by a few isolated groups with no real power to change society or public policy. And as long as tobacco use continued to be perceived as an issue of minor importance, a strong policy response was unlikely.

The dominance of doctors in tobacco control organizations kept the focus mainly on health, with little attention to the nonhealth dimensions of the epidemic such as the direct and indirect costs of health care, including lost earnings. Tobacco control efforts mostly concentrated on school programs and the organization of rallies and other small-scale events on World No Tobacco Day. The emphasis on talking to schoolchildren without taking other steps to address adult tobacco use may even have unintentionally attracted young people to using tobacco. In any case, the unsophisticated tobacco control messages were no match for glossy, attractive tobacco advertisements, particularly those of BAT.

One of the pioneer organizations involved in tobacco control was ADHUNIK, founded in 1987 by National Professor Nurul Islam.[1]

---

1. "National Professor" is an honorific title conferred by the government.

ADHUNIK representatives held many seminars and press conferences, published information in newspapers, appeared on television, printed information about tobacco and Islam for distribution to Muslim religious leaders, and contributed to the syllabus for class 8 in Bangladeshi schools. They also succeeded in making the president's residence a non-smoking establishment (ADHUNIK 1988).

Some other organizations have worked on tobacco control for many years. Among them are

- The Bangladesh Cancer Society, which has long attempted to raise concern about the issue of tobacco use, mostly through school campaigns and programs highlighting the connection between tobacco and cancer. In 1995 the Cancer Society also printed a booklet that discussed the economics of tobacco in Bangladesh, including the viability of alternative crops (Ahmad 1995).
- MANAS, started in the 1990s by Dr. Arup Ratan Chowdhury, a well-known dentist and singer. Its main activity is conducting school campaigns and seminars, as well as presenting programs on television.
- The National Non-Smokers' Forum, founded in 1986—the first anti-tobacco organization in Bangladesh. It publishes a quarterly newsletter and undertakes various public relations activities such as running seminars and workshops and printing informational materials.

These organizations are still active, both independently and in collaboration with BATA, whose founding is described in the next section.[2]

Before 1999 most of these groups focused on awareness-raising activities, particularly on health and for school-age children. What was missing was a determined effort to urge the government to pass strong tobacco control legislation, as well as the information and research needed to demonstrate the multisectoral nature of the problems of tobacco use.

The Catalyst for Change

It was a specific marketing campaign by BAT that finally provided the impetus for a concerted and courageous effort by tobacco control advocates. Even though advocates had become used to the flashy, sophisticated

---

2. ADHUNIK and the Bangladesh Cancer Society played an active role when BATA was first formed. As a result of internal politics, ADHUNIK is no longer active in BATA, and the Cancer Society has formally withdrawn. In April 2001 ADHUNIK announced that it was forming its own alliance, the Coalition Against Tobacco (CAT).

cigarette advertisements on television, in newspapers, and on billboards throughout the country, BAT's Voyage of Discovery campaign in the summer of 1999 was startling. The idea of sailing a yacht carrying the John Player Gold Leaf brand logo to 17 countries in 177 days caught people's imagination. The excitement was enhanced by the choice of the port of Chittagong as the final destination.

Alarming as were the billboards, newspaper advertisements, and cigarette display stands embossed with the Voyage colors and its slogan "Go for the Adventure," more worrisome were the lengthy and highly sophisticated television advertisements on the national TV station, Bangladesh TeleVision (BTV). Despite a law prohibiting BTV from carrying tobacco advertisements, the station repeatedly broadcast advertisements for the Voyage. This blatant disregard for national law in pursuit of profit, and the national fervor about the Voyage, caused a wave of unprecedented concern about tobacco control. But the concern was mixed with a sense of despair, as there seemed little that tobacco control advocates could do in the face of the wealth and power of BAT.

In July 1999 Work for a Better Bangladesh (WBB), a new organization devoted to tobacco control and urban environmental issues, organized a meeting to discuss possible responses to the Voyage campaign. Although only one other organization, the National Non-Smokers' Forum, was represented at this first meeting, the WBB was not deterred. What these tobacco control advocates lacked in wealth and power, they more than made up for in persistence. WBB staff contacted other organizations that might be interested—groups working on drug problems, development, consumer issues, and women's issues—and continued to organize meetings. Gradually attendance increased, and BATA was born. The WBB, on behalf of BATA, organized a press conference at which dignitaries, including Nurul Islam, founding president of ADHUNIK, spoke. At a seminar organized by BATA, a range of organizations presented their views, and barrister Tania Amir of the firm Law Associates offered her ideas on legal remedies that were unlikely to succeed but were worth trying in the absence of other possibilities. (Amir later founded Law and Society Trust, Bangladesh—LSTB—a member organization of BATA.)

Besides attracting advocates to the cause, BATA faced the challenge of raising funds for its activities. Most of the groups in BATA were small and had limited funds, and the larger organizations faced administrative difficulties in committing a significant amount of money for advocacy work. To overcome the hurdle, all of the organizations involved agreed to contribute small amounts; PATH Canada provided further financial assistance.[3] With a total of US$3,000—in marked contrast to BAT's annual advertising budget of US$3.3 million—the groups moved forward with their strategy.

From September to November 1999, BATA members conducted a series of activities, with different organizations taking the lead for different events. The president of the WBB, Saifuddin Ahmed, flew to Chittagong and looked through the docking permits for the Voyage campaign. He discovered that the yacht had not obtained proper permission, having applied to dock on a visit rather than for commercial purposes. BATA members designed and posted in cities all over the country "Sinking Boat" posters comparing the Voyage to the British colonization of Bangladesh. They also organized a bicycle rally from Dhaka to Chittagong, human chains in Dhaka and Chittagong, a press conference, and other events. Tania Amir of LSTB, barrister Omar Sadat of ADHUNIK, and several other individuals involved in BATA filed a petition with the High Court seeking a stop to the promotional activities planned on the yacht's arrival. BATA members made their voices heard, and their message was clear: the Voyage was not about adventure, glamour, or sophistication but about the efforts of a rich transnational company to hook poor Bangladeshis on expensive cigarettes.

The boat docked in Chittagong on November 21, 1999, one day after its expected arrival date. The mayor of Chittagong attended an event to greet the yacht, declaring that while cigarettes are dangerous to health, he welcomed foreign investment in Bangladesh. Almost simultaneously, the High Court issued its decision: a stay order on all promotional activities of the yacht. The concerts and other events were canceled, tickets were refunded, and a small notice was published in the paper explaining the occurrence. The yacht sailed away quietly a few days later.

When the case was reheard a few months later, the lawyer for BAT—one of the highest-ranking people in the opposition party—defended the Voyage as being not an advertisement for cigarettes but merely a generic promotion. His statement was challenged by barristers Omar Sadat and Tania Amir, who argued that the defense was absurd and pointed out the dangers of tobacco and the need for strong controls. With no laws to back up the argument against advertising (a law banning advertisements had been blocked in Parliament years before), Amir utilized the constitutional guarantee of right to life to support the case, arguing that the promotion of a product that causes serious disease and death is not consistent with the government's mandate to support health and life.

---

3. PATH Canada (the acronym stands for Programme for Appropriate Technology in Health) is an NGO based in Ottawa.

The judge agreed with the arguments of Sadat and Amir and issued a decision that urged the respondents, including the government, to:

- Ban production of tobacco leaf in phases, give subsidies to tobacco farmers to produce other agricultural products, and help tobacco workers find other jobs through such means as providing vocational training
- Restrict permission and licenses for establishing tobacco factories and direct the owners to switch to other products in phases, compensating them if necessary
- Persuade owners of tobacco factories not to continue with production of tobacco products beyond a reasonable time by banning such production
- Close down the bidi factories in phases and restrict the harvesting of tobacco to produce bidis
- Discontinue advertising of tobacco products and forbid any show or program that propagates smoking beyond the period of the existing contract or agreement
- Prohibit import of tobacco "within a reasonable period" and in the meantime impose a heavy import tax; require all imports to print a statutory warning legibly in bold type in Bengali
- Ban any promotional ventures such as the Voyage of Discovery
- Ban smoking in public places.[4]

The High Court had made an astonishingly strong ruling in favor of tobacco control, and BATA had been born out of the ashes of the Voyage campaign (Efroymson 2000a).

Power in Numbers: The Importance of BATA

Despite the victory in the High Court, the Voyage has not, in fact, disappeared from Bangladesh. Billboards still display the yacht, with the slogan changed to say "Follow the World Adventure." But more than just the billboards serve as a reminder of the yacht's eventful visit to Bangladesh. BATA, the alliance that was formed to fight against the Voyage, is the legacy and continues in its efforts to achieve better tobacco control policies for Bangladesh.

---

4. Bangladesh High Court Division Hearing on Writ Petition No. 1825 of 1999 and Writ Petition No. 4521 of 1999 in the Matter of an Application under Article 102 of the Constitution of the People's Republic of Bangladesh; summary available on the BATA Website, <http://bata.globalink.org>.

A key aspect of Bangladesh's new approach to tobacco control has been to widen the debate beyond health and enlist advocates from fields other than medicine (Efroymson 2000b). Although doctors around the world have achieved important successes in tobacco control, the exclusion of other groups has limited the effectiveness of advocacy efforts. People from fields such as law, consumer rights, and development work can bring different perspectives to the debate and additional tools to the advocacy movement, along with, potentially, a keener focus on law and policy.

Tobacco-related diseases are not considered a health priority in Bangladesh, and to focus exclusively on them would have essentially guaranteed failure in bringing about any major changes in tobacco control laws and policies. Rather than attempt to quantify the disease and death caused by tobacco, BATA focused instead on an issue of much more immediate relevance: malnutrition. As mentioned earlier, the poor of Bangladesh—as in many other countries—are much more likely to smoke than the wealthy, and the money they spend on tobacco, if used instead to purchase food, could make a significant difference in their children's nutritional status.

BATA now has 270 diverse organizations around the country in its network, as well as an international advisory board. In addition to MANAS and the National Non-Smokers' Forum, the following organizations are members:

- *Body Against Destructive Social Activities, Bangladesh (BADSA).* An antidrug organization, founded in 1994, that regularly organizes rallies and other events to highlight the problem of tobacco use in Bangladesh.
- *Consumers' Association of Bangladesh (CAB).* As part of its mandate to protect consumers, addresses the issue of tobacco as the most dangerous of all consumer products.
- *Dhaka Ahsania Mission.* Works in many sectors and has conducted many activities in tobacco control, including organizing (jointly with the LSTB) a discussion meeting on tobacco control law; persuading the Bangladesh Postal Department to produce a stamp and other materials celebrating World No Tobacco Day; organizing discussion meetings throughout the country; running a program to establish smoke-free schools; and printing and distributing stickers and posters.
- *Ghas Phul Nodi.* An antidrug organization; conducts various activities to draw attention to the problems of tobacco use.
- *Institute of Allergy and Clinical Immunology, Bangladesh (IACIB).* One of BATA's newest members; recently carried out a survey of ricksha pullers and their tobacco use habits and is conducting awareness programs.

- *Law and Society Trust, Bangladesh (LSTB)*. A key party in obtaining the High Court decision against BAT. Tania Amir of the LSTB has been active in the Intergovernmental Negotiating Body (INB) meetings for the Framework Convention on Tobacco Control (FCTC) and in revising legislation for submission to the government. She is a member of the law-drafting committee of the Ministry of Health.
- *MANOBIK (Madok Drabya-O-Nesha Birodi Council [Antidrug Council])*. An antidrug association that has recently taken on tobacco control as a major issue. Its activities include a sit-in protest in front of the National Press Club in favor of higher taxes on tobacco products and organization of rallies and discussion meetings.
- *Pratyasha*. An antidrug organization that conducts awareness campaigns on tobacco.
- *Welfare Association for Cancer Care (WACC)*. Currently focuses on involving more organizations in addressing women's and children's issues with respect to tobacco control. It has produced various materials addressing women's tobacco use, as well as a book on tobacco and cancer that highlights the human face of tobacco-related illness.
- *Work for a Better Bangladesh (WBB)*. The WBB, as BATA's secretariat, plays a key role in coordinating BATA events. It has conducted a series of tobacco control training workshops throughout the country. It coproduced, with PATH Canada, the "Hungry for Tobacco" report and two PATH Canada publications: a how-to guide for tobacco control and a guide to tobacco control law. The WBB has issued and is distributing, through BATA, a booklet of advice on quitting smoking, and it has produced various leaflets, stickers, and posters. Saifuddin Ahmed, WBB president and coordinator for BATA, has attended INB meetings, is active in the Framework Convention Alliance (a coalition of NGOs working for a strong FCTC), and sits on the law-drafting committee of the Ministry of Health.
- *Young Power in Social Action (YPSA)*. Based in Chittagong; had a critical role in organizing events to protest the landing of the Voyage of Discovery yacht in Chittagong port. With the WBB, it also organized a workshop in Chittagong, and it is active in encouraging local organizations to work on tobacco control.

The BATA member organizations listed here are NGOs registered with the government of Bangladesh. With the exception of the YPSA, all are based in Dhaka. Most are small organizations with a flexible structure that facilitates their involvement in the politically sensitive area of advocacy.

BATA's mission is to:

- Contribute to the health and well-being of Bangladeshis by reducing tobacco consumption

- Reduce the damage to health, the environment, households, and the national economy from tobacco consumption
- Educate the public and policymakers about the dangers of tobacco
- Help strengthen the nation's tobacco control policies and legislation
- Conduct research to learn more about tobacco use and its effects, particularly its economic impact
- Raise awareness among development organizations about the importance of tobacco control and encourage more groups to become involved
- Continue to be a strong, united force in tobacco control locally, nationally, and internationally.

The alliance has been active since its inception in leading and coordinating activities pertaining to education, awareness raising, training, advocacy, research, and coordination with government and NGOs on both the national and the international levels. These activities are an example of how NGOs can influence policy and build coalitions, as long as the members are willing to suspend an interest in exercising control and assuming leadership in order to work cooperatively. The following are just some examples of activities that BATA has championed since its founding in 1999:

- *Advocacy.* BATA has regularly held events calling for legislative changes, including a signature campaign in favor of nonsmoking carriages on trains and protests calling for higher tobacco taxes and an end to tobacco advertising. BATA is also urging the government to negotiate for and sign a strong Framework Convention on Tobacco Control.
- *Draft legislation.* After compiling laws from various countries, BATA helped draft a comprehensive tobacco control law which, as of March 2003, was still being discussed in parliamentary committees and is yet to be voted on by Parliament. The draft law bans advertising (except at point of sale), mandates pictorial warnings on cigarette packs, and prohibits smoking in many public places. BATA is working to strengthen the provisions and to ensure that the law is not weakened by Parliament.
- *Public education.* BATA members produce a range of materials, including posters, stickers, and pamphlets, to educate the public about the dangers to health, economics, and appearance from tobacco use and about how to quit smoking.
- *Public mobilization.* BATA encourages the public to take a stand against tobacco promotion and use. Mobilization activities include rallies and marches for the WHO's South-East Asian Anti-Tobacco (SEAAT) Flame for Freedom from Tobacco campaign in which, in 2000, a torch symbolizing the tobacco control movement traveled throughout South and

Southeast Asia. BATA has also held workshops, seminars, and press conferences on tobacco control themes.

- *Research.* BATA has conducted studies on the effect of tobacco use on poverty and has carried out research on demand for a smoke-free bus service. It has also run an analysis of BAT's "Youth Smoking Prevention Campaign," which included use of focus groups and a questionnaire.
- *International activities.* BATA has attended and made presentations at various international workshops and conferences, including regional meetings in India and Thailand, the People's Health Assembly, various WHO meetings, and the 11th World Conference on Tobacco or Health. Fifteen of its member organizations have made submissions to the WHO expressing support for a strong FCTC, and BATA is an active participant in the Framework Convention Alliance.

By broadening the base of support for tobacco control, BATA hopes to build a much stronger movement for tobacco control advocacy. With that in mind, the WBB, with financial support from the American Cancer Society and technical support from PATH Canada, is holding a series of workshops around the country for NGOs and the media on tobacco control. The workshops emphasize that tobacco is a multisectoral issue, one that touches on the environment, poverty, human rights, religion, and many other areas, as well as health. In the workshops the participants, mostly from small local NGOs, engage in small-group discussions to plan activities and create work plans. The WBB hopes in the future to provide small grants for these NGOs to encourage them to put some of their ideas into practice.

Tobacco control policy cannot be successfully formulated or implemented unless a broad base of NGOs around the country actively supports it. Effective support for a large NGO network is in turn contingent upon raising awareness among NGOs about the importance of tobacco control and their capacity to become effective advocates. In BATA's case, technical and financial support from American and Canadian agencies has been essential in enhancing the capacity of local NGOs to support the government and promote good policies for tobacco control.

The Politics of Policymaking

Bangladesh's democracy does not always operate smoothly. Rather than discussing issues in Parliament, the opposition party sometimes stages walkouts and then protests if decisions are made in members' absence. The most common form of protest is a *hartal* (general strike), in which a party or a coalition of parties asks people to stay home, usually from dawn to dusk. Reported cases of corruption and bribery within the government system further undermine the democratic process. These characteristics, coupled with the influence that tobacco companies wield, make tobacco control efforts difficult.

Despite all the vagaries of Bangladeshi politics, the government holds most of the solutions to the problem of tobacco use. Without strong laws and high tobacco taxes, there is little that organizations and individuals can do. This should not be used as an excuse to accept defeat; rather, it should be a reminder to everyone working in the field of tobacco control of the importance of continuing advocacy work.

Bangladesh's existing laws on tobacco control are weak. Advertising is banned on state-controlled media (BTV and radio) but is allowed everywhere else, including on local private and satellite television stations, in newspapers and magazines, and on billboards. Sponsorship of rock concerts by BAT (e.g., Benson & Hedges Star Search) is common, and despite the claim that youths under 18 are not admitted, no such rules appear to be followed (WBB and PATH Canada 2001). In addition, airing the programs on television effectively guarantees a young audience. One national daily newspaper, *Bhorer Kagoj*, voluntarily refuses to run tobacco advertisements (Simpson 1998), but other newspapers frequently run half-page, full-color advertisements for cigarettes. Billboards, storefront signs, cigarette display cases, and other forms of advertising are widespread throughout the country.

Smoking is banned in hospitals and some other premises, but these prohibitions are largely ignored. Operators of many air-conditioned buses and some owners of air-conditioned restaurants voluntarily forbid smoking. Biman, the national airline, prohibited smoking on domestic flights years ago, and in April 2001 it extended the ban to all international flights.

Warnings on tobacco products are limited to cigarette packs and consist of one weak statement, in Bengali and in small type, on the side of the pack. None of the other tobacco products available on the market are required to carry a warning.

The government is currently in the lengthy process of revising its tobacco control laws and drafting new ones. Pressure to do so came largely from the High Court's decision following the Voyage of Discovery case. If the new draft law under consideration is passed in its present form, it will be an enormous improvement and will provide a strong legislative base for better tobacco control in Bangladesh. Advocates continue to work to convince policymakers of the need for a comprehensive ban on promotions, strong and clearly visible warnings on all tobacco products, and protection of nonsmokers, among other measures.

BATA has developed a close working relationship with the government on the basis of simple principles appropriate to the Bangladeshi cultural environment, such as working with the government, rather than against it, and providing assistance to the government in carrying out its programs where possible. BATA members generally regard confrontational tactics as counterproductive in dealing with the government. In their view, the key to success in Bangladesh lies in maintaining a strong, close working relationship with the government and thus being able to form a constructive relationship with policymakers—an essential ingredient of effective tobacco control policies. Such a relationship does not preclude criticizing government policies or advocating strongly for change; rather, it involves a constructive attitude toward working with policymakers, based on mutual respect.

BATA tries to focus on providing services to the government—for example, designing stickers and posters and helping to organize government events. Where necessary, this includes providing services gratis and without taking credit. In return, the government is open to collaboration. Although this process means extra work for tobacco advocates, the payoff can be significant in developing and maintaining a strong relationship with the government.

Some of the ways in which BATA has sought to provide support for the government include:

- Organizing activities for WHO's Flame for Freedom from Tobacco campaign.
- Designing posters and organizing rallies for World No Tobacco Day.
- Briefing the government on the Framework Convention on Tobacco Control. This gave delegates the information they needed to participate in meetings and allowed BATA to present its view of the proposed language for the FCTC during the government negotiations.

The relationship between BATA and the government has been close and successful enough that BATA received the WHO's Tobacco Free World Award in 2001 at the recommendation of the government. In addition, two members of BATA—Tania Amir of the LSTB and Saifuddin Ahmed of the WBB—have been invited to sit on the Health Ministry's law-drafting committee and to participate directly in the process of drafting new legislation. In some respects BATA members now serve as a liaison between other BATA organizations and the government, soliciting ideas from members on what should go into the laws and what language should be used. The battle will not end with the passage of new laws: BATA members will also have a critical role to play in monitoring the behavior of the tobacco companies and ensuring enforcement of the laws.

Lessons Learned

Despite the progress that has been made, challenges remain. Among them are funding, the struggle to build the political will necessary for change and to establish tobacco control as a priority for the country, the construction of lasting alliances, and the continuing strength of the opposition. But important lessons have been learned in each of these areas.

Obtaining Funds

Important work such as advocacy for new laws can be done even with limited funding. Some of the strongest laws in other countries were passed when tobacco control movements had relatively little funding, as in South Africa and Thailand. But although ample funding does not guarantee success, it is difficult to do the work with *no* funding; critical tasks such as law enforcement and surveillance of the epidemic to measure progress can be expensive. Certain assets that are taken for granted in developed countries—a steady power supply, phone lines, computers, e-mail and Web access, and a good command of English—are in short supply in many developing countries. Such comparatively simple matters as finding basic information to back up a proposal for new laws, a space in which to hold meetings, and the money to print documents can be major obstacles. Lack of full-time staff devoted to tobacco control—and with access to resources—can seriously undermine efforts. From the perspective of tobacco control advocates, the ideal source of funding is a dedicated tax on tobacco, but advocacy groups need immediate funding to sustain the (perhaps lengthy) lobbying effort needed to get such a tax passed. Large organizations that have sufficient funds to conduct the work may shy away from advocacy, preferring less controversial areas such as school-based programs.

One way of overcoming lack of funds is through partnerships with local NGOs or with institutions in developed countries. To help provide at least minimal operating funds, PATH Canada offered the WBB some startup funding, shared office space, and, perhaps more important, ongoing technical input. PATH Canada's support enabled the WBB to focus on tobacco control work, including the building of BATA, rather than on seeking funds. The relationship also gave the WBB the assurance that small, necessary expenses could be met, such as those involved in holding a press conference and establishing computer and e-mail links for global networking. The technical assistance has been valuable in gathering evidence to support arguments for tobacco control. It enabled the WBB to provide the essential foundation and minimum operating costs for BATA, with other organizations contributing some funds and large amounts of time and expertise.

Having created an excellent track record in its first year of work, BATA was able to gain supplementary funding in the following forms:

- Three small one-year grants from the American Cancer Society to three BATA member organizations—the LSTB, to support legal advocacy; the Welfare Association for Cancer Care, to work on issues affecting women and children; and the WBB, to strengthen BATA through divisional workshops and printed materials
- A two-year grant from the Canadian International Development Agency (CIDA) to PATH Canada, the WBB, and BATA to develop and print materials, hold workshops, develop the capacity of WBB and BATA staff, and design and air counteradvertising.

In addition to these specific grants, BATA members have received funding from the WHO, the Rockefeller Foundation, the Canadian Cancer Society, and other groups to attend workshops, meetings, and conferences. Because dependence on external funding is a concern, BATA is seeking to increase contributions from its member organizations and to finance some of its publications by accepting advertising.

Much work can be done with little money if resources are used wisely. Writing letters, holding meetings, organizing public demonstrations, and talking to politicians cost little. Rather than waiting for funds to materialize, it is best to make a start, utilizing existing resources. If the work is successful, it will be easier to find funding in the future.

Creating Political Will and Working with the Media

It is often said that policy change cannot occur without political will. This statement seems to imply that political will is something innate rather than created—a dangerously passive approach to advocacy. Although that may sometimes be the case, a critical part of tobacco control is to create the will to make the changes. And in a democratic government, this often means convincing politicians that they will gain more votes if they are seen to support tobacco control.

How does one go about generating political will?

- *Educate and involve the public.* A public unaware of the problems associated with tobacco use and of the role the tobacco industry plays in blocking legislation will not put pressure on politicians for change. The public needs to know not only that tobacco is harmful but also what role the tobacco industry plays in opposing policies designed to reduce tobacco use. Involving the public includes taking the lead in activities such as letter-writing campaigns, petitions, and public demonstrations.

- *Educate politicians.* Politicians need to know how the tobacco industry may be trying to manipulate them through public relations activities and lobbying (e.g., suggesting that taxes be lowered to reduce smuggling when in fact the tobacco company itself has been shown to be involved in smuggling in several court cases). They need to understand the implications of tobacco use on health and the economy. And they need to know that activists will not keep quiet. Well-intentioned but ill-informed politicians can be educated to support tobacco control, and others can be shamed into doing so.
- *Show politicians that there is strong public demand for tobacco control.* Creating visible support for the issue—through public demonstrations, editorials, letters to the editor, and so on—can help persuade politicians that they will gain more by doing as the public wants than by pleasing their friends in the industry.

The media are critical to the creation of political will. Given the low budgets of most tobacco control programs around the world, the use of free media coverage is essential. One of the successes of tobacco control work in Bangladesh has been the ability to gain media attention. Activities have included:

- Holding press conferences.
- Inviting the media to seminars and workshops.
- Organizing rallies, human chains, and other protests, often in front of the National Press Club.
- Writing letters to the editor.
- Holding discussions with the newspaper *Bhorer Kagoj* that led to the publication of color messages about tobacco every day during the month of May, free of charge.
- Maintaining positive relations with the press. For instance, the *Economic Times,* a weekly newspaper on economic issues, frequently carries news releases provided by BATA.

It is possible that the willingness of the media to report on tobacco control topics, including the dangers of tobacco use, is in inverse proportion to the amount of income they gain from tobacco advertisements, although no study on this has been done in Bangladesh. The authors' subjective observation is that newspapers such as *Bhorer Kagoj,* with no tobacco advertisements, and *The Observer,* with only sporadic ones, devote more attention to tobacco-related problems than do newspapers that regularly run tobacco advertisements.

The media in many countries gain significant income from tobacco advertising, but there are always some individuals and institutions that are willing to help prevent disease and death from tobacco use, that envision a more effective role for the government in tobacco control, and that are prepared to provide support gratis. Building relationships with the press often pays off in free media coverage. We do not know what is possible until we try.

Competing Priorities

In many low-income countries there is a general feeling that tobacco control is an issue for rich countries that have the "luxury" of being able to worry about chronic diseases, while low-income countries have to concentrate on infectious disease, malnutrition, access to clean water, and the like. Framing the tobacco problem only in terms of cancer, or even only in terms of health, adds to this perception. Talking about the number of deaths likely to result from tobacco use can be ineffective, as many such deaths are likely to occur late in life. Where life expectancy is low, mortality from cancer and heart disease is not likely to be considered a priority, no matter how significant it may in fact be.

While never forgetting that tobacco is primarily a health issue, tobacco control advocates in Bangladesh have tried to stress that the health problems arise not only from disease but also from the opportunity costs involved in spending money on an addictive and harmful substance rather than on food or other basic needs. The argument is most appropriate when applied to transnational tobacco companies whose products are essentially unaffordable for most of the population yet are so widely advertised that they are likely to become aspirational goods, even at the cost of a large portion of family income. Repositioning tobacco use as an issue of poverty, nutrition, and human rights can gain the attention and support needed to deal with an entirely preventable epidemic.

It is important to be innovative in framing the tobacco control issue and to use concepts appropriate to the setting. In some areas the focus might best be on the environmental damage resulting from tobacco cultivation and curing; in others, on the labor issues involved in tobacco production. Tobacco control advocates should be flexible enough to present the issue in a way that broadens support and to obtain or develop the knowledge base on which to build their efforts and claims.

Maintaining a Strong Alliance

Alliances can be powerful tools, but they are often fraught with problems. It can be difficult to maintain a balance between attending to the organizational and relationship issues that have to be addressed to keep the alliance functioning and staying focused on the actual work of tobacco control. Bangladesh has experienced mixed success in this area: although BATA is strong and continues to grow, it has not been able to maintain the involvement of all the key players.

Working within a coalition has many advantages:

- The coalition can draw on the strengths of individual members, giving it access to a base of skills, experience, and connections that would be hard to find in any single organization.
- A coalition increases the number of voices speaking out and thus the level of attention to the issue.
- A coalition can be a forum for sharing ideas and communicating about individual actions so that even when joint organizing does not occur, work is more coordinated and groups do not unnecessarily duplicate each other's efforts.
- A coalition can, when it functions well, be an energizing force, where individual members gain ideas and motivation from each other and all face the work with greater eagerness.

But maintaining a strong and active coalition is difficult. Challenges can arise if individuals focus on personal gains and prestige more than on group plans or institutional objectives, if there is conflict over the best approach to shared work, and if personal conflicts or animosity arise. In such cases, creating smaller working groups or committees may be the way to continue building the group's effectiveness.

In Bangladesh the formation of an alliance was critical to the successes achieved. A balance is always needed between the administrative, organizational, and personal tasks needed to keep individual members satisfied and a focus on the work at hand. There is no such thing as a "perfect" coalition, but if the group can achieve more than was previously possible, without impossibly high inputs of time and other resources, then it can be described as successful. While the building of an alliance or coalition is one way to increase effectiveness in tobacco control, by no means should it come at an excessive cost in money, time, or energy.

Standing Up to the Opposition

The task of tobacco control often—and understandably—appears daunting. What can a few individuals or organizations working in the interest of public health do when faced with the power of one or several transnational tobacco companies, with their enormous financial resources and political connections? At least David and Goliath were standing on the same field; the tobacco industry may have access to lawmakers and other officials that tobacco control advocates can only guess at and wish for.

It is unrealistic to expect that the task will be simple. There will always be times of discouragement. It is important to keep a sense of perspective and to remember that even in the countries that boast the greatest successes in tobacco control, about a quarter of the population still smokes; in many other countries, the percentage is far higher and continues to rise.

Every time a tobacco company launches a new public relations campaign, or a government cuts tobacco taxes or refuses to pass new legislation or passes legislation drafted by the tobacco industry itself, there is a need for advocates to take stock. Yes, the tobacco industry is a powerful adversary, and yes, the companies have vast financial resources, but they are also trading in a deadly and addictive product that most of the population does not consume and that most addicted users wish they could stop using. The victories achieved by tobacco control advocates and policymakers are almost always hard-fought. There are plenty of setbacks along the way, and a long way farther to go, but however great the power of might, even greater is the power of right.

A powerful opponent can sometimes provide motivation. BATA was formed during the struggle against BAT over the Voyage of Discovery, and other work was inspired by BAT's launch of its "Youth Smoking Prevention Campaign." Policymakers and advocates, working together, will be able to curb BAT's ability to advertise, thus narrowing the gap between the tobacco industry's reach and BATA's. The only sure path to defeat is to accept it without a struggle.

Conclusion

Most of the story of tobacco control in Bangladesh is still unwritten, and events continue to unfold. It remains to be seen whether the tobacco control movement will be sufficiently powerful and proactive to counter industry tactics and persuade the government to take strong measures to control tobacco. The tobacco industry is a mighty force in Bangladesh, as elsewhere, and it will be difficult to maintain a spotlight on tobacco in the face of so many competing causes of disease and ill health. But if the progress made over the past few years is any indication of the future, the many organizations and individuals working for tobacco control in Bangladesh have good reason to be optimistic.

References

ADHUNIK (Amra Dhumpan Nibaron Kori). 1988. "Proceedings of the First National Seminar on Tobacco and Smoking, 1988, Dhaka, Bangladesh." Dhaka.

Ahmad, M. 1995. "Tobacco and the Economy of Bangladesh." Keynote speech delivered on World No Tobacco Day, May 1995. Bangladesh Cancer Society, Dhaka.

Bangladesh Bureau of Statistics. 1996. *Prevalence of Smoking in Bangladesh.* Dhaka.

———. 1998a. *Household Expenditure Survey 1995–96.* Dhaka.

———. 1998b. *Foreign Trade Statistics of Bangladesh 1997–1998.* Dhaka.

———. 1999. *Statistical Pocketbook Bangladesh 1998.* Dhaka.

BAT (British American Tobacco). 1998. "Reports & Accounts 1998." Dhaka.

———. 2000. "Code of Conduct." Dhaka.

BATA (Bangladesh Anti-Tobacco Alliance). 2001. *Mukhapotro Newsletter,* April–June (in Bengali). Dhaka.

Corrao, M. A., G. E. Guindon, N. Sharma, and D. F. Shookoohi, eds. 2000. "Tobacco Control Country Profiles." American Cancer Society, Atlanta, Ga.

Efroymson, D. 2000a. "Bangladesh: Voyage of Disdain Sunk without Trace." *Tobacco Control* 9 (2): 130–31. Available at <http://tc.bmjjournals.com/cgi/content/full/9/2/129b>.

———. 2000b. "BATA Battles BAT in Bangladesh." *Global Health & Environment Monitor* 8 (2).

Efroymson, D., S. Ahmed, J. Townsend, S. Alam, A. Dey, R. Shah, B. Dhar, A. Sujon, K. Ahmed, and O. Rahman. 2001. "Hungry for Tobacco: An Analysis of the Economic Impact of Tobacco Consumption on the Poor in Bangladesh." *Tobacco Control* 10 (3): 212–17. Available at <http://tc.bmjjournals.com/cgi/content/full/10/3/212>.

Haq, N. 2001. Oral presentation at Tobacco Control Workshop, April 2001, Chittagong, Bangladesh. Work for a Better Bangladesh, Dhaka.

Shaha, R., B. Dhar, and D. Efroymson. 2000. "Satellite Television Advertising in Bangladesh." Presentation at the 11th World Conference on Tobacco or Health, 2000, Chicago, Ill.

Simpson, D. 1998. "Bangladesh: Not a Cigarette Paper." *Tobacco Control* 7 (3): 228–29. Available at <http://tc.bmjjournals.com/cgi/content/full/7/3/227c>.

UNICEF (United Nations Children's Fund). 1998. *The State of the World's Children 1998.* New York: Oxford University Press.

———. 2000. "Child Work in the Bidi Industry." Dhaka.

WBB (Work for a Better Bangladesh) and PATH Canada. 2001. "BAT's Youth Smoking Prevention Program: What Are the Actual Goals?" Dhaka.

WHO (World Health Organization). 1997. *Tobacco or Health: A Global Status Report.* Geneva.

World Bank. 1999. *Curbing the Epidemic: Governments and the Economics of Tobacco Control.* Development in Practice series. Washington, D.C.

3
Government Leadership in Tobacco Control: Brazil's Experience

Luisa M. da Costa e Silva Goldfarb

A broad national network of dedicated activists helped achieve Brazil's success in tobacco control. Thousands of committed individuals have worked together and have enlisted the support of politicians, religious leaders, and the media to increase public awareness of the hazards of tobacco use and limit the influence of the tobacco industry. Their voluntary and professional efforts have made Brazil a world leader in tobacco control.

This case study describes the creation and consolidation of Brazil's National Tobacco Control Program (NTCP) at the National Cancer Institute (INCA). It emphasizes the strategic decisions that led to new laws, higher taxes, and educational programs.

The Scope of the Tobacco Problem in Brazil

Tobacco consumption in Brazil—as in other countries in Latin America—grew throughout the 1970s and 1980s, fueled by a significant increase in the proportion of females smoking (PAHO 1992; USDHHS 1992). By 1989, 30 percent of the population over the age of 15 smoked. Of Brazil's 30.6 million smokers, 18 million (59 percent) were male and 12.6 million (41 percent) were female (Ministry of Health and IBGE 1989).

In 1989, 2.742 million Brazilian children and adolescents age 5–19 smoked. Of these, 369,767 were between the ages of 10 and 14, and 2,341,151 were age 15–19. Among children younger than 10 years old, there were 30,531 smokers, 98 percent of them in rural areas (Ministry of Health and IBGE 1989). Surveys in 10 Brazilian state capital cities in 1987, 1989, 1993, and 1997 showed an increase in the percentage of school attenders age 10–18 using tobacco for the first time (Galduróz, Noto, and Carlini 1997: 130).

The same studies showed that first use of tobacco among girls increased between 1987 and 1997. By the 1997 survey, in 3 of the 10 state capitals studied—Porto Alegre, Rio de Janeiro, and São Paulo—first-use numbers for the 10–18 age group were higher for girls than for boys. In Curitiba, Salvador, and Recife there was no statistically significant difference between boys and girls in age of first use. The study concluded that the percentages of male and female smokers would soon be equal.

The data on young Brazilian smokers, in particular, raised the alarm. Studies have shown that 50 percent of those who try cigarettes for the first time as adolescents become adult smokers (Henningfield, Cohen, and Slade 1991; USDHHS 1994; WHO 1998). The data highlighted the urgent need for measures to reduce the number of young people who experiment with smoking.

Health and Environmental Effects of Tobacco Use and Production

An estimated 80,000 people die every year in Brazil from the effects of tobacco use (Silva and others 1998b: 71). Cardiovascular diseases are by far the biggest cause of death, accounting for 27.5 percent of all deaths, and cancers are in fourth place; both are strongly related to tobacco use (Ministry of Health 1999a; Duchiade 1995).

Added to the gloomy health data for smoking is the impact of tobacco production on people and the environment. Tobacco crops are grown with intensive use of chemicals: soil sterilizers, fertilizers, and pesticides that can all be highly toxic (Perez 1990). This means that both people and the environment—soil, water, air, and animals—have been systematically contaminated by chemicals for years. Brazil also suffers other negative effects of growing tobacco. The use of wood to feed 116,000 ovens to cure tobacco leaves has contributed to the loss of native forests in southern Brazil, which are now only 2 percent of their original extent (Quesada and others 1989; Lopes and others 1992).

Brazil's Tobacco Economy

Brazil is the biggest tobacco exporter and the third largest tobacco producer in the world. In 2000 it produced 595,000 metric tons of tobacco leaves and exported 341,000 tons, which brought in US$961.2 million in revenues (MDIC/SECEX 2001). The size of the tobacco industry in Brazil can also be measured by the 165,000 families (about 700,000 people) who make their living from growing tobacco and the 1.3 million more whose income indirectly derives from the tobacco industry (ABIFUMO 2000). Taking measures that could affect this economy requires considerable care.

Changing the tobacco economy may not be as difficult as it seems, however, because the Brazilian economy does not depend on tobacco production. Only 2.6 percent of all export earnings comes from tobacco. (By contrast, in Zimbabwe the percentage is 23 percent and in Malawi,

61 percent—World Bank 1999: 122.) Of course every job is important, but tobacco farmers represent only 0.44 of 1 percent of all full-time jobs in Brazil, and even if indirect employment is added, the tobacco industry's contribution to employment is small. Furthermore, if people stop smoking, they spend the money on other goods and services instead, and this generates new jobs across the economy.

As a tobacco exporter, Brazil must prepare for global changes in consumption. Tobacco controls are growing stronger around the world, and the industry is shifting its sources of supply. This could well lead to a drop in demand for Brazil's tobacco, and supply must adjust. The sooner that a tobacco-exporting economy such as Brazil begins to redirect investments away from tobacco, the quicker and better it will be able to adjust to future global consumption and trade patterns.

Given the environmental damage and health risks from tobacco, 41 percent of tobacco producers surveyed in southern Brazil said they would switch from tobacco to another crop if certain economic conditions existed, including the availability of good credit and a guarantee of a market for the new crop (Etges 1989). The results of this survey were reinforced at a meeting in 2001 of farmers, government officials, workers, and institutions interested in the fate of the tobacco economy. Farmers emphasized that they would need financial help to switch to alternative crops (Ministry of Health and others 2001).

Government Support for Tobacco

Farmers are only one part of the tobacco economy. Firms involved in manufacturing and selling tobacco products make up another powerful group. Vigorous lobbying by this industry has produced a level of government support out of proportion to the commodity's economic importance. Data show that since 1997, 22 percent of all resources from the National Program for Family-Run Agricultural Businesses (PRONAF) has been used for tobacco crops, particularly in the south, where 93 percent of tobacco production is concentrated (BACEN 1999; Ministry of Health 2000a). Aiming to reduce this percentage, the Brazilian Central Bank has forbidden the use of PRONAF funds to finance tobacco production in partnership with or through "integration" with the tobacco industry (Resolution 002833, April 25, 2001). Individual tobacco growers are still eligible for these funds, but they lose their eligibility if the tobacco industry acts as an intermediary for them or if they have any direct association with tobacco companies.

The Beginnings of Tobacco Control in Brazil

As long ago as the early 1970s, some Brazilians were worried about the harmful effects of tobacco. But actions to control its use were limited by pressure from the industry and by lack of knowledge among health professionals, politicians, and the general public.

The first attempts at tobacco control took place in several different areas: Bahia, Paraná, Espírito Santo, Rio Grande do Sul, São Paulo, and Rio de Janeiro. The main players, and the driving force behind these attempts, were health professionals—mostly physicians—motivated by information from international publications. Some of the original tobacco control advocates are still active. Dr. J. Rosemberg of Sorocaba Medical School deserves special mention because of his inspiring example. At the age of 93, he is the president of the Coordinating Committee for Tobacco Control in Brazil (CCCTB) and is still speaking up about tobacco.

In 1977 the National Cancer Association drew up an action plan to control tobacco use. The following year, as a spinoff of the plan, the association organized Anti-Tobacco Use Week and launched Rosemberg's book *Tobacco Use: A Public Health Issue.* Two years later, acting on a proposal by the Brazilian Cancer Society, the Brazilian Medical Association organized local committees to give talks to physicians about the effects of tobacco use. They also pressed to have the subject added to the curricula of medical and paramedical schools and placed on the agenda of medical congresses around the country.

In 1979 the First Symposium on Tuberculosis took place in Salvador, Bahia state. The resulting "Salvador Letter" contained information and warnings about the harmful health effects of tobacco use (Rosemberg 1987). The letter also provided the first estimate of mortality related to tobacco use in Brazil: 100,000 per year. (Later, this figure was revised downward.) The letter recommended a two-pronged preventive approach to controlling tobacco use through education and legislation. In April 1980 the First Brazilian Conference against Tobacco Use was held in Vitória, Espírito Santo state, and produced a similar document, the "Vitória Letter" (Rosemberg 1987).

Growing awareness of the dangers of tobacco use increased public support for tobacco control activities. Politicians in some states recognized the strength of this support and added tobacco control to their political agendas. The state of Paraná, for example, organized the first Strike Against Tobacco Use and established the statewide Day Against Tobacco (Law 7,419, 1980). During the strike, students collected tolls from passing motorists to raise funds for the campaign, educational handouts were distributed, and nonprofit organizations provided funding to support the effort.

In the early 1980s countries in the region created the Latin American Coordinating Committee for Tobacco Control (CLACCTA) through an initiative of the U.S. Centers for Disease Control and Prevention (CDC) and the American Cancer Society. CLACCTA's first president was the late Dr. Mario Rigatto, a very active professional from Rio Grande do Sul and one of the pioneers in Brazilian tobacco control.

Brazilian tobacco control efforts evolved slowly until 1985, when the federal government began participating in the process. Health Minister Waldir Arcoverde established a commission to write a national tobacco control action plan for the ministry. The commission worked quietly for more than six months, avoiding attention from the industry and its lobbyists. Brazil's first Action Plan for Tobacco Control was completed in 1986.

An important element in the plan was the involvement of the National Health Foundation (FUNASA) of the Ministry of Health. FUNASA's existing national network for tuberculosis control became the distribution system for information about the harmful health effects of tobacco, with pneumologists Germano Gherardi, José do Vale Feitosa, and Miguel Aiub Hijjar playing key roles.

In June 1986 Federal Law 7,488/86 created the National Day Against Tobacco (August 29) and reserved the week prior to the day for national events related to the issue. That law, although weak, was a great step forward in Brazilian tobacco control legislation.

Gaining Momentum: The National Tobacco Control Program

Brazilian tobacco control efforts reached a turning point in 1987, when the National Tobacco Control Program (NTCP) was established. The head of the chronic degenerative disease unit in the Ministry of Health, Geniberto Paiva Campos, provided the needed support and political status to launch tobacco activities under the program through INCA, which designated Vera Luiza da Costa e Silva as its representative on the program. Between 1987 and 1989 the group in charge of the NTCP was limited to a few professionals who worked under INCA's coordination but were based in different departments of the Ministry of Health. NTCP's first strategic action was to identify health technicians in the state health secretariats to act as NTCP's state coordinators and to be responsible for delivering the program in their states.

Also in 1987, the Ministry of Health established the Advisory Board on Tobacco Use Control, and the first National Day Against Tobacco was celebrated. This was the first time that the Brazilian people were officially given information about the damage caused by tobacco and the importance of reducing its use.

Business Joins In

Businesses were involved early in tobacco control efforts. The law that created the National Day Against Tobacco appealed to businesses by instituting an honors certificate awarded by the Ministries of Health and

Labor to companies that attained certain standards such as workplace smoking bans, restricted smoking areas, and educational programs. The participation of business greatly benefited the program because the companies' actions provided examples for others to follow. In the first eight years only a few companies received certificates, but since 1996 the numbers have grown, and the system has become a success. The Central Bank (Banco do Brasil) deserves special recognition because of its participation in the plan right from the beginning.

Banco do Brasil has contributed enormously to the program. It has been a role model for other companies and institutions through its occupational health initiatives, including tobacco control, and its support for sports and "healthy" events such as swimming, jumping, running, dancing, and athletic competitions known as Largue o Cigarro Correndo (Running Away from Cigarettes). In the 1990s these competitions were taken to 600 cities where the bank's Workers' Athletic Association (AABB) had branches. This increased the NTCP's visibility around the country and spread information about the harmful health effects of tobacco to the general public.

Later, as a part of World No Tobacco Day, coordinated by the World Health Organization (WHO), the NTCP's coordinating body extended the honors certificate awards to individuals who supported the government's campaign against tobacco. People in the media, writers, actors, lawyers, teachers, and athletes have received certificates. The awards have attracted considerable public attention and wide media coverage—so much so that the president and the health minister are increasingly seen at these celebrations.

Support Grows

Public campaigns against tobacco grew in importance as people's understanding of tobacco's harmful health effects increased. Between 1987 and 1989 a variety of activities boosted public awareness.

- In 1988 Ministry of Health Act 490 required cigarette packs to display the warning "The Ministry of Health advises: smoking causes damage to health."
- A survey showed that 70 percent of children questioned lived in a home where at least one person smoked (Silva 1987). This statistic was widely discussed in the media.
- Some 70,000 students from 16 states took part in the antitobacco Children's Slogan and Drawing Contest.
- Radio and TV campaigns on the effects of secondhand smoke were launched, with great impact on public opinion.

- A children's comic magazine, *Stop Smoking Around Me,* by a major Brazilian comic book artist and featuring a well-known female hero, was published.
- Four posters designed by another Brazilian comic book artist and targeted at different population groups were distributed around the country. Ten years later, one of these posters appeared on the cover of the international journal *Tobacco Control,* published by the British Medical Journal Publishing Group.

Efforts Stall and Then Resume

Tobacco control efforts abruptly stalled in 1990 when the NTCP was taken from INCA and transferred to Brasília. This shift brought the program to a halt. At that time, the author became part of the INCA team, which continued its involvement in tobacco control at an institutional level. At the end of 1992 Health Minister Adib Jatene moved the NTCP back to INCA. The INCA team was delighted: the minister had the political will needed to carry on the program. Vera da Costa e Silva was once again in charge of the NTCP. In 1993 INCA restarted the program with a technical coordinating team that consisted of Vera da Costa e Silva, Tânia M. Cavalcante, Tereza P. Feitosa, and the author.

The team pushed hard to make up for lost time. It ran its first capacity-building workshop in 73 health units in Rio de Janeiro—a first step in taking the NTCP to local health units. In addition, an annual evaluation and planning meeting was held at which 14 of Brazil's 27 states were represented. Much work still needed to be done to cover all the states.

That same year, NTCP staff participated in the Annual Seminar on Alternative Crops organized by the Catholic Church. They debated with tobacco growers and agrotechnicians in southern Brazil, the heart of tobacco production in the country. As a result of that work, today 1,000 families grow alternative crops such as corn and beans instead of tobacco.

The NTCP was gaining ground, and demand for action was growing. Team members felt that they had to take advantage of the favorable political climate created by a succession of ministers who were at least not against tobacco control action, if not explicitly for it. Above all, they wanted to act while Marcos Moraes was director of INCA. He strongly supported public health initiatives and was interested in moving tobacco control forward.

The team recognized the need to consolidate the process of creating partnerships and attracting qualified people with varied professional backgrounds to the program. With this goal in mind, in 1994 INCA organized the First National Congress on Tobacco Use, with the support of FUNASA and the CCCTB. Over 400 people attended the meeting, including politicians, Catholic Church leaders, lawyers, teachers, physicians, nurses, psychologists, and media professionals. During the congress, the WHO awarded INCA the Tobacco or Health Prize for its work on tobacco control.

As a result of the congress, a partnership among the main health professional associations began. Meetings were held in 1996 and 1999. In 2000, 21 associations met and produced the *Consensus on the Treatment of Tobacco Users*, which INCA published in 2001 and is distributing to health professionals across the country. The *Consensus* was the first document published in Brazil that provided a technical guide for health professionals who want to help smokers quit (Ministry of Health, INCA, and CONPREV 2001a).

Throughout the 1990s, tobacco control events became stronger and more frequent, with the yearly celebrations of World No Tobacco Day (May 31) and the National Day Against Tobacco (August 29). The National Day Against Tobacco, which promotes a link between sports, arts, and not smoking, has become more and more popular across the country. The NTCP team at INCA coordinates the central production of all publications and advertisements with the aim of improving communication through the use of a single message and image.

Restricting Tobacco Advertising and Promotion

At the end of 1994 the NTCP team handed the health minister a daring initiative—a proposed bill banning all direct and indirect advertising and promotion of tobacco products. The bill would also require that packages of tobacco products display the Ministry of Health's six rotating health warnings.

When the proposed bill arrived in Congress, an intense debate about its constitutionality erupted between the government on one side and the tobacco industry and its allies (advertising professionals and representatives of television and radio advertisers) on the other. The industry and its allies argued that the bill was a crime against freedom of information. The NTCP team welcomed the debate because it provided additional publicity about the harmful effects of tobacco use.

The outcome was weaker legislation (Law 477/1995) that merely restricted tobacco advertising to the hours between 9 p.m. and 6 a.m. and included less assertive warnings on cigarette packs. For example, the word "may" was added to the warning about heart attacks so that instead of stating "Tobacco causes heart attacks," it read "Tobacco may cause heart attacks."

Tobacco control measures in the 1990s were not as strong as advocates would have liked, but they seem to have had an impact on cigarette consumption. Decreases in real prices in 1990–91 and between 1992 and 1994

Figure 3.1. Trends in Cigarette Consumption and Real Prices, Brazil, 1983–94

Index (1983=100)

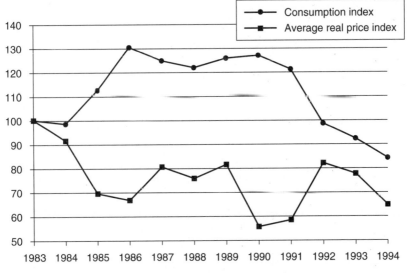

Source: Silva and others (1999).

should have led to an increase in consumption, as had happened between 1983 and 1986 (a period of extremely high inflation). Figure 3.1 shows that consumption fell in the late 1980s and early 1990s, suggesting that the usual effect of lower prices was counteracted by other factors such as health warnings on cigarette packs, limits on indoor smoking, and restrictions on tobacco advertising (Silva and others 1999).

Economic Measures Considered

In 1995 the NTCP team decided that it was time to consider adding economic measures to existing tobacco control efforts. Published evidence from other countries indicated that an increase in prices would lead to a decrease in tobacco consumption. Health Minister Adib Jatene ordered an econometric study to evaluate the impact of a price change on consumption and supply in Brazil. The study provided the NTCP team and other tobacco control players with the information needed to coax the financial and economic sector to work with them.

In the meantime, worried about the contents of tobacco products sold in Brazil, the NTCP team sent five samples of the most popular cigarette brands to Canada for content analysis. NTCP staff compared the results with limits for tar, nicotine, and other components set by countries where the contents of tobacco products were controlled. The Brazilian cigarettes exceeded most limits.

Both the econometric study and the content analysis proved valuable in 1999 when they were used to support the inclusion of tobacco in the list of substances regulated by the National Sanitary Vigilance Agency (ANVISA), the Brazilian counterpart of the U.S. Food and Drug Administration. Both studies and their results were summarized in *Brazilian Cigarettes: Analyses and Proposals to Reduce Consumption* (Silva and others 1999).

The States Become Involved

The NTCP team knew that its activities had to be improved and expanded if the program were to succeed. These efforts depended, as usual, on political decisions; policymakers and decisionmakers had to be committed to the program. Accordingly, at the end of 1995 the NTCP team proposed that the health secretaries of all the Brazilian states be invited to the NTCP's annual evaluation and planning meeting. The meeting, chaired by Health Minister Jatene, was held during the national meeting of the State Health Secretaries Council. It included the first appraisal of NTCP management in the states and a presentation of the program's needs for resources for local action.

This was a historic moment: tobacco control finally became part of the health agenda in all the states. An agreement was reached in which financial resources were transferred from the central to the local governments. Those resources could be used only for a work plan developed and assessed annually by the states and INCA together and supervised by INCA.

Implementing Decentralization

The increased involvement of the states reinforced the NTCP team's commitment to decentralization. To be successful, the program had to reach people across the country, but Brazil's huge area and large population created a challenge. The NTCP team took advantage of the existing network of the Ministry of Health Management System to develop a decentralized program for tobacco activities.

In 1996 NTCP team members gave management training courses to staff from all 27 state health secretariats and 300 municipal health secretariats. This helped develop a large, well-trained national workforce at the local level. That 300 municipalities were willing to allocate funds and to send their staff for training was an indication of the demand for the courses and of commitment across the country. The relatively large numbers of people involved helped persuade policymakers and decisionmakers to allocate federal funds to build capacity for local NTCP staff and other agents. Since 1997, training courses have been held all over the country.

Two books have been written about the experience: *Basis for the Implementation of a Tobacco Control Program* (Goldfarb and others 1996) and *Practical Guidelines for the Implementation of a Tobacco Control Program* (Silva and others 1998a). The local health secretariats use these books to prepare courses and train staff. In addition, the WHO Tobacco Free Initiative, now coordinated by Vera L. da Costa e Silva, uses these texts and the methodology they describe for similar actions in other countries around the world.

INCA Becomes a WHO Collaborating Center

Recognizing the need to encourage new people to take part in the NTCP, INCA supported the state of Ceará in northeastern Brazil when, in 1996, the state hosted the Second National Congress on Tobacco Use. This congress had twice as many participants as the first one, held in 1994, and it established the basis for a National System for the Evaluation and Surveillance of Tobacco Control. Since 1996, the congress has been held in different regions. Each congress produces a document, "Final Recommendations," that establishes the basis for further action on tobacco control in Brazil.

At the 1996 congress INCA's director, Marcos Moraes, announced an expansion of the responsibilities of NTCP staff. Within their ambit would be the National Coordination of Tobacco Control and Primary Cancer Prevention (CONTAPP), which included the NTCP and other prevention programs for cancer risk factors.

At the end of 1996 Brazil was designated a WHO Collaborating Center for the Tobacco or Health Program. With this move, INCA had achieved both national and international importance: it was now responsible for providing information on the WHO Tobacco or Health Program to Brazil and beyond—to Latin America, and to Portuguese- and Spanish-speaking countries all over the world.

The national coordination bulletin *Tobacco News* became a key tool for INCA in fulfilling this mandate. Published in Portuguese since 1992 and in English and in Spanish since 1994, *Tobacco News* was distributed to 100 institutions and individuals around the world and to 19 Latin American countries, in addition to 10,000 subscribers in Brazil. In 1996 its scope was widened to include other risk factors. It was also used to set out the guidelines for the Collaborating Center's activities. Another publication, *Data and Facts,* was created in 1999 to communicate news about tobacco issues in Brazil and around the world, and about the NTCP's actions during the negotiations for the WHO Framework Convention on Tobacco Control (FCTC).

In 1996 INCA began the first of a series of research projects to support its tobacco control efforts. The first research study evaluated a pilot project on educational interventions in four schools in Rio de Janeiro city. The pilot project was designed to provide experience and to test materials for the National School-Based Health Knowledge (Saber Saúde) Program. In 2000 an analysis of the project's research results was presented in a public health master's degree thesis, which demonstrated that the intervention significantly reduced tobacco experimentation among students (Goldfarb 2000).

More International Involvement

From November 1996 on, 12 professionals were on the staff of CONTAPP (which included the NTCP). In addition to the four physicians who had worked there from the beginning and another physician, they included a lawyer, a teacher, a chemist, a psychologist, a nutritionist, a nurse, and an epidemiologist. Attracted by the dimensions of the NTCP and the availability of NTCP/INCA facilities and staff support, two major events took place in Rio de Janeiro in 1998: the annual meeting of CLACCTA and the Seminar for an Agenda on Tobacco Control Priority Research for Latin America and the Caribbean Islands.

The first event brought together representatives from 19 countries and from the CDC, the Pan American Health Organization (PAHO), the WHO, and the American Heart Association. CONTAPP staff took the opportunity to present Brazil's tobacco control activities and plans in detail. This led to discussions of the possibility of using the Brazilian experience to develop pilot studies in other countries throughout the region.

The second event, supported and chaired by Research for International Tobacco Control (RITC)—a secretariat of the International Development Research Centre (IDRC) in Canada—brought together researchers from a variety of institutions. As a result of their participation, many of these institutions adopted tobacco control as a priority action item (RITC 1998).

Research Continues

Research on tobacco-related topics continued on several fronts. In 1998 the "Study on the Impact of Tobacco Use on Death by Heart Attack among Women Aged between 35 and 59 Years in Rio de Janeiro" was the subject of a doctoral thesis in public health that showed a positive association between tobacco use and myocardial infarction among women in the studied population (Silva 1999).

To expand research efforts, the Ministry of Health, through INCA, began developing research links with universities. In 1998 a partnership with Johns Hopkins University in the United States was signed to carry out a study on smoking behavior, passive smoking, and the determining factors for nicotine levels in saliva in Rio de Janeiro. The study was completed at the end of 2002. Preliminary data show a drop in smoking prevalence in Rio among adults (age 15 years and older) from 30 percent in 1989 to 21 percent in 2002. The reduction is strongest among the 16–24 age group and is larger for men than for women. Of the smokers interviewed, 85 percent were aware that passive smoke causes harm; 53 percent supported a total smoking ban in restaurants; 70 percent supported a ban on all advertising; and 76 percent supported a ban on sports sponsorship by the tobacco industry.

With a view to stimulating research, the NTCP team began reserving part of its budget for studies within the states to evaluate local educational interventions in schools, health units, and workplaces. This initiative has had limited success so far because it has been difficult to find qualified professionals at the local level to conduct the evaluations.

In 1999 NTCP staff broadened the scope of research to investigate other health issues in addition to tobacco. Experts from different areas were invited to formulate questions for the National Household Survey on Risk Behavior and Related Morbidity from Noncommunicable Diseases, funded by the World Bank and by two institutions associated with the Brazilian Ministry of Health: FUNASA and the National Centre for Epidemiology. Data collection began in 2002, and preliminary data will be available in 2004.

Also in 1999, the NTCP tobacco control pilot project in workplaces was evaluated and described in a master's thesis in occupational health (Feitosa 1999). This study supported the findings of previous research showing a positive relationship between educational interventions and reduction in tobacco use. It formed the basis for the NTCP's workplace programs.

In 2000 another study evaluated the Tobacco-Free INCA Program, designed to make INCA's buildings tobacco free. This study, which also showed a positive relationship between educational interventions and reduction of tobacco use, formed the basis for NTCP programs in health service units (Ministry of Health 2000b).

Support for strengthening the program's outreach to health professionals came from a master's thesis in public health on physicians' attitudes toward tobacco use, tobacco users, and their efforts to stop smoking (Cavalcante 2001). Physicians' attitudes and preconceptions about tobacco use, its health effects, and its addictiveness were shown to affect their support for and use of training and related materials.

The commitment to research continues. Important surveys were carried out in 2002: the National Survey on Tobacco Use among students, sponsored by a partnership between the Brazilian states and INCA/Ministry of Health, and the CDC/PAHO/WHO Global Youth Tobacco Use Survey in 13 Brazilian municipalities (1 funded by PAHO and the WHO, 5 by INCA, and the rest by the Brazilian Health Ministry and by state health secretaries).

Political Will Brings Increased Support

With the CLACCTA and IDRC events in Rio de Janeiro and the ongoing national activities, 1998 had been an intense year, but it still had a surprise in store. In December INCA's new director, Jacob Kliegerman, transferred early cancer detection to the NTCP team. Already in charge of programs for other cancer risk factors, this small team now had to balance its expanded responsibilities with those of the NTCP. Vera L. da Costa e Silva became the general coordinator of all prevention and detection programs, and the author took over coordination of risk factor prevention, in which the NTCP was involved.

The NTCP team members recognized that the time was right for greater action: they had physical facilities, were highly motivated, and continued to have the support of INCA's director. Above all, they had the health minister, José Serra, on their side. Serra was more than supportive: he became NTCP's leader and canvassed the president for his support as well.

Stronger Laws on Tobacco

From 1998 on, the framework of laws controlling tobacco and tobacco use broadened as a result of Serra's efforts (Ministry of Health, INCA, and CONPREV 2001d, 2001e). The first was Ministry of Health Ruling 2,818 in 1998, which banned smoking in the ministry building. A crucial next step was the approval in January 1999 of Federal Law 9,782, which established the ANVISA. With the creation of this agency, Brazil became a world leader in regulating and controlling the production, content, and advertising of tobacco products.

Also in 1999, Ministry of Health Ruling 695 mandated new, more assertive warnings to be published on cigarette packages. Two phrases were particularly striking:

- "Nicotine is a drug and causes addiction"—which represented a major victory against the industry
- "Smoking causes sexual impotence"—which put Brazil, only the second country in the world to adopt this warning, in the forefront of anti-tobacco action.

Next, ANVISA Resolution 320/99, requiring annual registry of tobacco products and reporting by the industry, was proposed. Companies would be required to pay a fee for each brand they produced. The money would have been used for funding tobacco control initiatives such as the Laboratory for Tobacco Analysis and the Centre for Clinical Studies on Nicotine Addition in INCA. This resolution was later replaced by Resolution 105.

The National Commission on Tobacco Use

In August 1999 Decree 3,136 created the National Commission on Tobacco Use (NCTU) to prepare Brazil for the coming world negotiations on the FCTC. The ministries represented on the commission are Inland Revenue, Health, Education, Development, Industry and Trade, Work Relations and Employment, Agriculture and Supply, Foreign Affairs, and Justice. Each minister nominates a representative. The president of the commission is the health minister, and the executive secretary is from INCA. By involving all these ministries—not only the Ministry of Health—the NTCP became a stronger program, with many ministries contributing to a common tobacco control effort, supported and implemented by states and municipalities across the nation.

Since its establishment, the NCTU has listened to many sectors of society, including tobacco proponents, to gather as much information as possible to support Brazilian actions at home and abroad. Its agenda includes important tobacco control issues within Brazil, such as a provisional measure to ban tobacco vending machines, which make it much easier for children and teenagers to buy cigarettes. One way that the tobacco industry tries to increase tobacco consumption is to make buying tobacco products as easy as possible.

The NCTU has held regular meetings to analyze its white paper for the FCTC that establishes the basis for the Brazilian position at meetings of the Intergovernmental Negotiating Body. It has also met with the Brazilian Tobacco Growers Association (AFUBRA), at that group's request, to discuss the growers' concerns about the FCTC (Ministry of Health INCA, and CONPREV 2001f).

In August 2000 the NCTU held the first public hearing on the FCTC. The hearing was designed both to inform the public and to receive input about Brazil's participation in the FCTC. Over 15 days, 30 institutions and interested individuals, including representatives from tobacco-related business, presented their interventions in favor of or against the FCTC/WHO document.

Swift Action and Strong Support: A Legislative Victory

Studies carried out abroad have confirmed the effectiveness of a comprehensive ban on tobacco product advertising in reducing tobacco consumption, especially among young people (Saffer 2000). In 2000 Brazilian society was ready to take this step, and the Ministry of Health decided to present an antitobacco bill to the Congress. The NTCP team knew that dealing with the tobacco industry would be a tough task. The industry had reacted fiercely whenever faced with restrictive legislation in other countries. Experiences such as the rejection by the U.S. Congress of proposed changes to legislation in 1988 suggested that rapid action would be the best way to get changes through.

Information on the new tobacco control strategy had to be provided quickly to key individuals and to the Brazilian people. The NTCP team focused on preparing to neutralize industry's attempts to interfere with the planned legislation. In May 2000 the health minister sent to Congress Bill 3,156, which would limit the advertising of tobacco products to the point of sale only. The action had begun.

Canvassing Public Support

To gain public support for the new bill, the Ministry of Health released the television movie *Traficante* (*Trafficker*), together with outdoor display advertisements and advertisements in the main Brazilian magazines. The campaign had enormous public impact. The movie showed the correlation between nicotine consumption and use of other drugs, and the similarity between drug dealers and the tobacco industry. At the same time, the ministry sponsored the exhibition *Seeing through the Smoke*, designed to attract public attention to the tobacco issue, promote discussion, and inform people, especially teenagers. The exhibition included publicity films, sculptures, videos, photos, and interactive installations in São Paulo, Brasília, and Rio de Janeiro.

Soon afterward, the Ministry of Health released the movie *Jornalista* (*Journalist*), in which a real person, a journalist, talked about his legs being amputated because of thrombosis caused by his dependence on tobacco.

The ministry's bold actions stirred enormous public interest. The press followed the issue closely and interviewed NTCP staff, INCA's director, and the health minister many times in the months before Congress voted on the bill.

To assess the campaign's impact, people in 100 municipalities were surveyed about the movie *Traficante*; 97 percent approved of it. In a national sample, 73 percent said they knew of the government's campaign against smoking, and 94 percent approved of the comparison between tobacco and drugs. For the movie *Jornalista*, public recall was almost 90 percent, one of the highest ever for a government prevention campaign (Ministry of Health and ASCOM 2000).

The industry reacted noisily, saying that it was surprised both by the government's action and by the content of the bill and that the law was too radical. It looked to advertising agencies and the public for support, and it lobbied members of Congress to include alcohol in the law. Health Minister Serra responded quickly by saying that those who wanted alcohol included in the law should be considered tobacco industry lobbyists. That was enough to defuse any attempt by members of Congress to support the countercampaign.

The Importance of Partnerships

The government now moved to enlist broad support by developing a contact network of 3,000 institutions. Information was sent out through the Internet, and handouts (similar to those produced by the European Union) were distributed that spelled out why tobacco advertising and sponsorship should be prohibited. INCA's Internet site included a discussion space that received about 250 comments and queries every month. E-mail addresses for members of Congress were publicized, and citizens sent them thousands of messages.

An interesting partnership was set up with the nongovernmental organization (NGO) Rede de Desenvolvimento Humano (REDEH), a collection of 5,000 pro-woman and citizen organizations. About 350 community radio stations belonging to CEMINA, a member of REDEH, aired spots warning about health damage from tobacco use and giving information on the proposed law.

The Brazilian Societies of Cardiology and Pediatrics, the Federal Medical Council, the Federal Council of Dentists, the Federal Nutrition Council, and the Brazilian Medical Academy all showed their support for the law by making public statements on its urgency and importance. Many international institutions also supported the law because of Brazil's position as a major tobacco producer and exporter and because of its potential to serve as an example to other countries.

Industry Action

Meanwhile, the tobacco industry and advertising agencies stepped up their actions. Tobacco proponents said they were puzzled by the "sensationalistic and radical way" the government was dealing with the matter. They claimed that Brazil's constitution guaranteed freedom of commercial expression for the tobacco industry.

The industry sent letters to 1,400 radio stations and 200 television stations condemning the ban on tobacco advertising and claiming that "to forbid [advertising] is to deny freedom of expression, the right to information, and consumer's freedom of choice." They recommended that the media spread a message emphasizing freedom of creation and expression—the "oxygen of publicity."

The media generally tried to present both sides of the discussion. But not everyone in the media had the same clear understanding of what was at stake. One newspaper published a message favoring tobacco and stating that "the president of Souza Cruz [Brazil's major cigarette producer and the Brazilian arm of British American Tobacco] defends the freedom of the market and maintains that the government ought not to interfere in people's lives or force them to be happy, healthy, or good."

In response, the NTCP/INCA distributed to the media a statement saying, "There is no freedom without responsibility. Freedom to advertise cigarettes may be restricted constitutionally for health reasons, particularly because it concerns a product that kills half its consumers and uses misleading advertising messages."

To widen the focus, two public debates were organized before the Commission of Constitution and Justice and the Commission of Social Affairs in the Brazilian Senate. The debates between lobbyists on both sides revolved mainly around freedom of expression, but the economy was also a key element. AFUBRA made a brief presentation and asked questions.

As the controversy boiled, the industry promoted a new strategy to bypass the existing law that prohibited smoking indoors: "smokers' lounges," with comfortable armchairs and complex air conditioning systems that were supposed to extract smoke and clean the air. (Considerable evidence shows that these air conditioning systems are not effective in protecting health; see Tobacco Free Kids 2001.) The promotion of smokers' lounges used images that associated smoking with a comfortable lifestyle.

On December 13, 2000, the tobacco control bill passed the Senate and the Chamber of Deputies, and on December 27 President Fernando Henrique Cardoso signed Law 10,167. Tobacco advertising now could appear only inside sales points. The industry reacted by trying to increase sales to compensate for those lost as a result of the new law. A new marketing strategy focused publicity at sales points, the only places it was still allowed. The industry increased the number of sales points and redesigned some of them as "tobacco shops," a new concept featuring attractive layouts and displays of antique and modern tobacco-related devices that appeal to art appreciation and curiosity. Sometimes a pipe maker demonstrates her craft. (Most pipe makers are women.)

The National Commission Deals with Rumors

The passage of Law 10,167 was a victory for tobacco control advocates, but it did not mean the battle was won. Skirmishes continued regarding many points. A crucial moment for the NCTU came in March 2001 during one of its routine meetings in southern Brazil. NCTU members planned to use the occasion to meet with 230 local people, including farmers, university teachers, agricultural technicians, tobacco industry workers, and members of syndicates, trade unions, and religious congregations, to discuss issues raised by the FCTC, particularly those related to alternative crops.

At first, the meeting did not go as planned, as rumors circulated that the government was going to ban tobacco growing. The International Tobacco Growers Association released a letter that presented an inaccurate analysis of the FCTC's intentions, causing great anxiety among workers in the region. At the time, the author was executive secretary of the NCTU, and she produced a series of papers to explain the government's position. The media became involved, and the event had greater repercussions than expected, but the message got through: Brazil was planning for a future of lower tobacco demand. Tobacco control measures around the world, following FCTC recommendations and actions, would cause demand for tobacco products to drop, and supply would be affected. Because Brazil is a major producer and exporter of tobacco, it had to anticipate this process so that adjustments could be as smooth as possible. The government was seeking ways of gradually substituting other crops for tobacco.

These arguments neutralized the rumors, and the farmers became less wary of the government representatives. They finally joined the discussion on what kind of help they needed and whether direct technical, financial, or operational support should be provided. The NCTU suggested that farmers, industry, and the government work together to answer these questions. The commission had turned its detractors' attacks to its advantage (Ministry of Health and others 2001).

More Tobacco Control Legislation

On March 28, 2001, ANVISA published Resolution 46. Among other provisions, the resolution sets maximum levels of tar, nicotine, and carbon monoxide allowed in cigarette smoke released by tobacco products sold in Brazil, which would bring them into line with European Union limits (table 3.1).

Resolution 46 also requires that every cigarette package carry information on the levels of these substances and the warning, "There are no safe levels for the consumption of these substances." The resolution was the first in the world to forbid the inclusion of any descriptive words or phrases such as "light," "ultra light," "low levels," "mild," "soft," "moderate levels," "high levels," or any others that might mislead consumers about the concentration of the listed substances. Through heavy lobbying, the industry succeeded in postponing the application of the law from 2001 to January 2002. At the time, the reason the delay was requested was

Table 3.1. Maximum Levels for Three Harmful Cigarette Smoke Ingredients, Brazil and the European Union (milligrams per cigarette)

	Tar	Nicotine	Carbon monoxide
Brazil			
January 2002	12	1	12
September 2002	10	1	10
European Union			
September 2000	10	1	10

Source: European Union, 2002.

unclear, but eventually it became obvious that the companies wanted the delay so they could launch new marketing campaigns using new package designs, colors, and layouts that would be associated with "light" cigarettes. After the prohibition came into effect, they could use these designs and colors to convey the idea without using the actual word "light."

On World No Tobacco Day, May 31, 2001, Health Minister Serra sent Congress another regulation toughening the legislation against tobacco advertising. Provisional measure 2,134/30 was signed and became effective in January 2002. Following Canada's example, the measure requires that the warnings on cigarette packages and advertisements be accompanied by a picture showing graphically what they mean.

At the end of that highly productive year, Resolution 105 was published. It required that all tobacco companies—manufacturers, importers, and exporters—be registered and submit annual reports to ANVISA on their tobacco products, the products' compositions, and sales and production levels.

Education: The Basis of the NTCP

The history of Brazil's tobacco control efforts shows how a steady buildup of commitment and action can lead to success. Together, education and legislation form the foundation of this achievement.

The "Cascade" System for Training

Early on in the struggle, NTCP team members recognized that they alone could not provide all the training needed to keep the program moving forward. The team therefore developed a cascade system to multiply its training efforts. The federal team (that is, the NTCP team) trains the staffs of state health and education secretariats, who then train staff from municipal health and education secretariats. They, in turn, train professional workers at workplaces—schools, health units, and so on—and these professionals use their training to reach out to the general public.

The NTCP training prepares local state and municipal agents for action at four activity levels. This staged set of actions, combined with the cascade training scheme, guarantees a network of capable people in the health and education systems. They work together within a framework that supports all the activities needed to advance tobacco control. The four levels are as follows:

Level 1
- Deciding on the local political, physical, and administrative structures for tobacco control initiatives
- Planning and evaluating local programs and activities
- Conducting public and media relations and keeping the tobacco control theme on the media agenda
- Giving general information talks on tobacco and the implications of its use and production
- Coordinating tobacco control activities at the local level
- Learning epidemiology basics

Level 2
- Within the local partnership of health and education secretariats, developing and coordinating continuous educational actions throughout the year across three community channels—schools, health units, and workplaces—with agents from the Family Health Program and the Community Agents for Health Program

Level 3
- In partnership with those responsible for epidemiology, carrying out surveys and research projects and implementing local initiatives of the National System of Evaluation and Surveillance on Tobacco

Level 4
- Encouraging the development of, proposing, and lobbying for adequate legislation and economic measures
- Providing techniques and support materials for the treatment of nicotine addiction

By 2002, teams in 26 states and the Federal District (Brasília) had been trained and were training others within levels 1 and 2. The work is being carried out in 3,150 cities—almost 60 percent of all cities in the country—

by 12,239 trained professionals (Ministry of Health, INCA, and CONPREV 2001b). Training for level 3 began in 2000 in all states and in Brasilia.

Level 4 training began in 2001 within the Help Your Patient Stop Smoking Program in five regions of the country. NTCP staff set priorities among routine counseling, group, and individual sessions according to the *Consensus on Treatment of Tobacco Users* (Ministry of Health, INCA, and CONPREV 2001a). To provide better support for these actions, the Tobacco Studies Laboratory Division at INCA's Centre for Clinical Studies on Nicotine Addiction (CCSNA) is studying the use of drugs to help people stop smoking. Through clinical trials, it will investigate the efficacy of nicotine replacement therapy, on its own and combined with behavioral interventions. The information from the studies will be used in deciding whether to subsidize public programs that support quitting smoking.

Also as part of level 4, at the beginning of 2001 a national plan for encouraging legislative strategies and actions was drawn up. The plan helps local advocates stimulate the creation of laws, promote lobbying, monitor legislation, and reinforce tobacco control legislation at the local level.

Tobacco Control Education in the Workplace, in Schools, and in Health Units

The most popular educational actions are the campaigns and celebrations, which are designed primarily to provoke, inform, and promote discussion. But these events are not enough to create the changes in attitudes, habits, and behavior needed to cut tobacco use. Continuous day-to-day actions are essential in health units, workplaces, and schools. In Brazil these actions are supported by experiences from the pilot studies mentioned earlier and compiled in the manuals *Implementing NTCP in Health Units, Implementing NTCP in Workplaces*, and *Implementing NTCP in Schools*.

The program in health units and workplaces aims first to achieve a tobacco-free environment through the Tobacco-Free Places Program. It then supports people who want to quit smoking through the Helping Your Patient Stop Smoking Program. These programs are led by health professionals, who are trained to become "multipliers." They implement the program inside their institutions and train others, who then train staff members and even clients. The training helps people understand their responsibilities as role models and how this relates to day-to-day behavior, particularly in health units. Respect for others is emphasized, with the aim of achieving a better quality of life for everybody.

In the workplace and in health units. In early 2002 the Tobacco-Free Places Program was already under way in 3,150 cities, and 1,042 companies were registered in the workplace program. Of these, 358 were taking action, and 83 had finished the process and were totally tobacco free.

Among health units, 530 were putting the program into practice (Ministry of Health, INCA, and CONPREV 2001b).

In schools. The statistics on first use of tobacco by children and adolescents at the beginning of this chapter highlight the need for antitobacco programs aimed at young people. The Saber Saúde health knowledge program was developed to meet this need. With its emphasis on the quality of life and health promotion, the program covers more than tobacco control issues; it also deals with alcohol, exposure to sun, diet, physical activity, sex, and occupational hazards.

Under the program, trained teachers develop classroom activities as they would for other subjects. The activities are related to the school's overall community life and to students' interests. Modules such as "The Smoke-Free School" can be adapted to each school. These program activities form themes across all disciplines, as required by the national curricula of the Ministry of Education: health, environment/ecology, ethics, citizenship/politics, and sexuality (Silva and others 1998a; Goldfarb and Monteiro 1999).

The Saber Saúde program has been welcomed by educators. National implementation began in 1998, and by 2002, 4,853 workers had been trained at the state education secretariats in 2,247 cities. By January 2002, 5,251 schools were registered in the program, and 2,983 of them had already trained between 70 and 100 percent of their teachers, for a total of 62,024 teachers. These teachers instruct 1,227,358 students in grades 1 to 8 (Ministry of Health, INCA, and CONPREV 2001c). Although this is not a huge number when compared with the total school population, it is still very encouraging. Many technical schools and universities are adapting the program for their own use, but the results of these initiatives are not yet available.

Legislative Action: Education's Partner

Education alone would be a slow road to success in tobacco control. Together, education and legislation move tobacco control efforts more rapidly toward their goal. In Brazil legislative actions take place in the wake of and in support of education initiatives. Education, in turn, supports legislation by teaching people about the law, why it exists, and how it is enforced. It also raises awareness that results in increased advocacy and support for tobacco control.

Legislation-related actions include:

• Creating and updating a database on tobacco legislation now in force and planned across the country
• Monitoring voting by political representatives

- Providing information to political representatives
- Researching technical information
- Providing advice and comments on proposed bills
- Lobbying.

The biggest challenge is informing people about the law and encouraging them both to obey it and to help enforce it. Helping people become better citizens involves changing attitudes and behavior.

Legislative actions, like educational ones, are carried out by the three levels of government: federal, state, and city (municipality). In 2000 alone the Congress sent 59 tobacco control bills to the NTCP for analysis. NTCP staff provide clear technical and political information to ensure that the proposed law supports public health interests. Feedback from the NTCP can result in changes being made to a bill or can even lead to its withdrawal.

At the state level, 72 laws regulating the publicity and consumption of tobacco have been passed, and at the municipal level, 331. Of the state and municipal laws, 73 percent have been approved since the NTCP's establishment (Ministry of Health, INCA, and CONPREV 2001d).

The Other Side of the Picture:
What Stimulates Consumption?

Brazilian tobacco advocates have made great progress in controlling tobacco use, despite the opposition of a huge international industry. The tobacco industry has invested an enormous amount of money in direct and indirect tobacco advertising to entice people to smoke. In 1994 US$6.6 billion was spent on direct tobacco publicity in Brazil (Nielsen Institute 1996).

Indirect tobacco advertising in Brazil and elsewhere in the world has associated tobacco use with sports, arts, music, popular artists, fashion shows, and celebrities by sponsoring events that involve these activities and people. Events related to education, ecology, and environmental protection have also become targets of tobacco sponsorship. In this way, the industry seeks to associate tobacco products with healthy activities to create a positive public image. For example, in 1999 tobacco company–sponsored programs Hortas Escolares (School Greenery Gardens) and Clube da Árvore (Tree Club) reached 3,700 rural schools, 120,000 students, and 5,000 teachers in the southern state of Santa Catarina. The programs praise the benefits of healthy foods and the importance of protecting the environment and preserving nature, and they teach students how to grow a school garden or make a reforestation camp (Souza Cruz 1999a).

A similar program by AFUBRA, A Vida é Verde (Life is Green), distributes seeds and teaches agriculture students how to plant them (AFUBRA 2000). In 1999 a partnership between AFUBRA, the Tobacco

Industry Syndicate (SINDIFUMO), and other institutions created a new program, O Futuro é Agora (The Future is Now), to train workers for jobs in agriculture.

Souza Cruz, a major Brazilian tobacco company, is one of the sponsors of the government education program Alfabetização Solidária (Support-ive Literacy Program) and has, through its own initiative, started the pro-gram Educar (Educate) to teach illiterate adults and provide technical training in agriculture. The company is also one of the sponsors of the environmental program Onda Azul (Blue Wave), which has been interna-tionally acknowledged and is led by the important Brazilian environmen-talist and popular music singer Gilberto Cil (Souza Cruz 1999b, 2001).

Another campaign, directly focused on younger people, produced advertisements with a double meaning: "Smoking after 18. That's Legal!" (Fumar só com 18 anos. Isso é legal!) and "Smoking? Only with an Iden-tity Card" (Fumar? Só com carteira de identidade) (Goldfarb and Mon-teiro 1999). The campaign presented itself as being supportive of the leg-islation that prohibits cigarette sales to teenagers younger than age 18, but in fact it was part of a worldwide campaign by the tobacco company Phillip Morris to reinforce the perception among young people that smok-ing is an adult activity—a prime reason for its attraction for youths.

All these publicity campaigns reveal the industry's keen interest in establishing a positive social image, particularly among young people. This interest coincided with the implementation of the NTCP's Saber Saúde program, which is aimed at teachers and students and focuses on health and the environment.

Low Prices Encourage Consumption

The low price of cigarettes in Brazil is another factor that has encouraged consumption. As shown in figure 3.2, Brazilian cigarette prices are rela-tively low by world standards, even though tax rates on cigarettes are rel-atively high (Sunley, Yurekli, and Chaloupka 2000: 421; Guindon, Tobin, and Yach 2002).

Studies in Europe, Canada, and the United States, as well as in Brazil, show that a 10 percent price rise causes a 3 to 6 percent decline in con-sumption. Among teenagers, the impact is even greater and may be as large as 14 percent in Brazil and 23 percent in Canada (Sweanor 1992; Townsend, Roderick, and Cooper 1994; European Union 1995; Silva and others 1999).

Silva and others (1999) presented data showing that cigarette con-sumption doubled between 1970 and 1980, from 72.7 to 142.7 billion units. It described the changes in annual per capita consumption of cigarettes in Brazil since 1980, which has gone through several fluctuations, decreasing and rising with changes in real prices and incomes.

Figure 3.2. Prices of Imported and Local-Brand Cigarettes, Selected Economies, March 2001

Pack of 20 at purchasing power parity

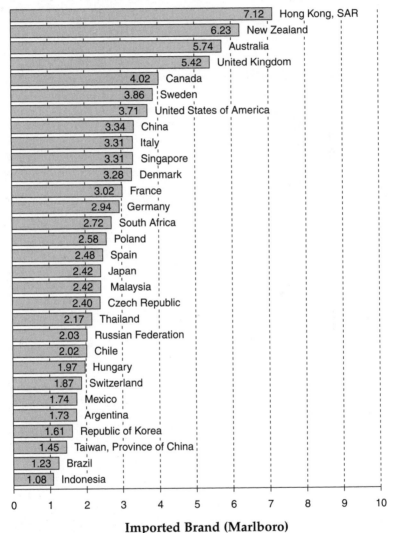

Imported Brand (Marlboro)

Figure 3.2. *(continued)*

Pack of 20 at purchasing power parity

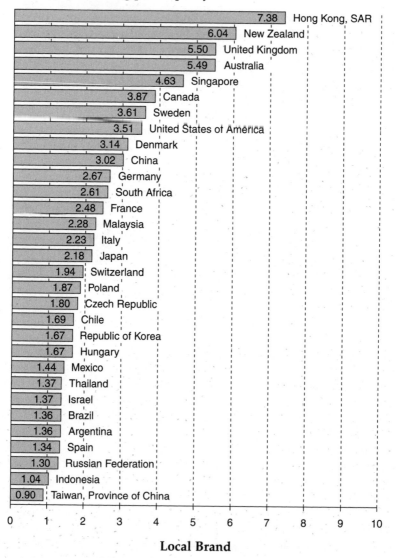

Local Brand

Note: The purchasing power parity index adjusts exchange rates for the relative cost of living in each economy. It allows a comparison of "affordability" rather than simply comparing prices.

Source: Guindon, Tobin, and Yach (2002). Reprinted from *Tobacco Control* 11 (1): 38 (2002), with permission of the BMJ Publishing Group.

Figure 3.3. Trends in Per Capita Cigarette Consumption by People Age 15 and Older, Brazil, 1980–99

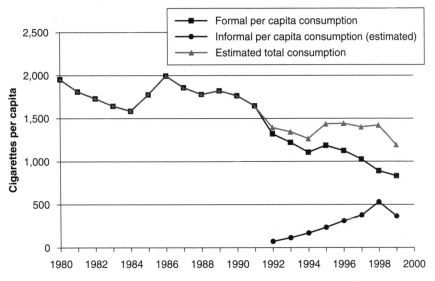

Source: Silva and others (1999).

Among people age 15 or over, annual per capita consumption decreased between 1980 and 1984 because of inflation that reduced purchasing power (see figure 3.3). Between 1985 and 1986, annual per capita consumption returned to pre-1980 levels as a result of a decrease in the real price of cigarettes. In 1987 the price rose again, and, as a consequence, per capita consumption dropped the next year. In 1989 this tendency was temporarily reversed by an increase in salaries, which had been frozen, but in 1990 per capita cigarette consumption dropped to 1,752. Official data implied that in 1992 the level was 1,305, but this figure hid the consumption of smuggled cigarettes and, on a lesser scale, counterfeit cigarettes, which were sold at lower prices and without any control. Actual consumption in 1992 was estimated at about 1,370 per capita. Until 1999 official consumption decreased and black market consumption increased, but total per capita consumption was thought to have remained stable at about 1,265. Even so, it was lower than the 1986 figure of about 1,950, leading to the conclusion that smuggling and the industry's massive investments in publicity had been counteracted by an effective tobacco control policy (Silva and others 1999; IBGE 2000; MDIC/SRF 2000).

The Role of Smuggling

One of the challenges of measuring and combating tobacco consumption in Brazil has been the impact of smuggled cigarettes, which come in mainly from neighboring countries. Some smuggling involves "round-tripping," in which cigarettes are legally exported but, instead of reaching their alleged export destination, are smuggled back into the exporting country. There are no official figures, but Inland Revenue's estimates for 1998 indicate that 58 billion cigarettes were sold on the black market. That figure corresponds to 40 percent of all cigarette consumption in Brazil. In 1999 around US$800 million was lost due to tax evasion related to cigarette smuggling (Ministry of Health 1999b; AFUBRA 2000; Ministry of Health, INCA, and CONPREV 2001d).

In an attempt to curb smuggling, the Inland Revenue Office in December 1998 imposed a 150 percent tax on cigarette exports to South American and Central American countries. Cigarette exports fell sharply, but soon afterward, exports of tobacco leaves rose (tobacco leaves are free of taxes). The number of cigarette-producing plants at sites just outside Brazil's borders increased (Ministry of Health, INCA, and CONPREV 2001d; Otta 2001). This shows that it is vitally important to monitor the tobacco industry's behavior so that smuggling can be understood and prevented. Resolution 105 was designed to provide such monitoring: as noted above, the industry must submit annual reports to ANVISA on their tobacco products, the products' composition, and their sales and production levels.

Lessons Learned

Brazil's experience with tobacco control demonstrates how a public health program can succeed despite economic and administrative challenges and strong resistance from commercial interests. The lessons to be drawn focus on the role of dedicated individuals and organizations in linking information, education, and legislation to create a potent force for change.

The key lessons from the Brazilian experience are as follows:

- *Develop and foster public commitment to tobacco control.* Without this commitment, coupled with strong leadership, the NTCP and other advocates could not have achieved as much as they have.
- *Use a decentralized strategy to get the message out.* Brazil benefited from a strategy based on trainers instructing other trainers so that the message could be spread across the country.
- *Seek political support from those in power.* Public commitment would accomplish little without the political will to sponsor legislation.

- *Participate in partnerships with all sectors of society:* professional associations (particularly those in the health sector), the media, politicians, well-known artists and sports people, and religious organizations. These partnerships, based on respect and accurate information, were a great help in the process. They provided another means of getting the message out and helped persuade government ministers and the president to support tobacco control efforts.
- *Carry out and support research.* Evaluations, prevalence surveys, econometric studies, opinion polls, political assessments, and other studies build a strong evidence base that allows sound decisions to be made and actions to be taken quickly.
- *Act quickly.* Speed is essential in developing and approving legislation and educational programs and improving them. Changes should arise from the interaction between education and legislation.
- *Do not give in to industry pressures,* no matter how innocuous the demands might seem. Agreements with the industry must be avoided; they only delay the adoption of new measures. There is not a second to be lost in this race.

References

ABIFUMO (Brazilian Tobacco Industry Association). 2000. *Tobacco Industry Profile* (in Portuguese). Brasília.

AFUBRA (Brazilian Tobacco Growers Association). 2000. *Brazilian Tobacco Annual Report* (in Portuguese). Santa Cruz do Sul.

BACEN (Central Bank of Brazil). 1999. "Rural Ordinary Operations Register" (in Portuguese). Brasília.

Cavalcante, T. M. 2001. "Physicians and Their Perceptions of Tobacco Use, Smokers and Smoking Cessation" (in Portuguese). Master's thesis. National Public Health School, Oswaldo Cruz Foundation (FIOCRUZ), Rio de Janeiro.

Duchiade, M. P. 1995. "Brazilian Population: A Moving Photo." In M. C. S. Minayo, ed., *Many Brazils: Health and Population in the 1980s* (in Portuguese). Rio de Janeiro: HUCITEC.

Etges, V. E. 1989. "Submission and Resistance: Gaucho Farmers and the Tobacco Industry" (in Portuguese). Master's thesis. São Paulo University.

European Union. 1995. "Tobacco Taxes in the European Union: How to Make Them Work for Health." Health Education Authority, London.

———. 2002. "Tough EU rules on manufacture, presentation and sale of tobacco products take effect." Press release DN: IP/02/1383. September 27. Brussels. Available at: <http://europa.eu.int/rapid/start/cgi/guesten.ksh?p_action. gettxt=gt&doc=IP/02/1383 I 0 I RAPID&lg=EN&display=>.

Feitosa, T. M. P. 1999. "Workplaces and Tobacco Use: Implementing a Tobacco Control Program in Companies" (in Portuguese). Master's thesis. Federal University of Rio de Janeiro.

Galduróz, F. J. C., A. R. Noto, and E. A. Carlini. 1997. "IV Survey on Drug Use among High School Students: Data from 10 Brazilian Capitals" (in Portuguese).

UFSP/CEBRID/EPM (Federal University of São Paulo/Brazilian Information Center on Psychotropic Drugs/Medical School of São Paulo and Psychobiology Department), São Paulo.

Goldfarb, L. M. C. S. 2000. "Evaluation of Tobacco and Other Risk Factors Control Program in Four Schools in Rio de Janeiro City" (in Portuguese). Master's thesis. National Public Health School, Oswaldo Cruz Foundation (FIOCRUZ), Rio de Janeiro.

Goldfarb, L. M. C. S., and A. M. F. C. Monteiro. 1999. "Implementing a School-Based Program for Tobacco Control and the Prevention of Other Cancer Risk Factors" (in Portuguese). Ministry of Health/INCA, Rio de Janeiro.

Goldfarb, L. M. C. S., A. M. F. C. Monteiro, and V. L. C. Silva. 1998. "Saber Saúde. Tobacco Use and the Prevention of Other Cancer Risk Factors. Guidelines with Proposals for Teachers" (in Portuguese). Ministry of Health/INCA, Rio de Janeiro.

Goldfarb, L. M. C. S., T. M. Cavalcante, V. L. C. Silva, T. P. Feitosa, and A. R. Abib. 1996. *Basis for the Implementation of a Tobacco Control Program* (in Portuguese). Rio de Janeiro: Ministry of Health/INCA.

Guindon, E., S. Tobin, and D. Yach. 2002. "Trends and Affordability of Cigarette Prices: Ample Room for Tax Increases and Related Health Gains." *Tobacco Control* 11 (1): 35–43. Available at <http://tc.bmjjournals.com/cgi/content/full/11/1/35>.

Henningfield, J. E., C. Cohen, and J. D. Slade. 1991. "Is Nicotine More Addictive Than Cocaine?" *British Journal of Addiction* 86 (5): 565–69.

IBGE (Brazilian Institute of Geography and Statistics). 2000. "CENSO/Population National Data" (in Portuguese). Rio de Janeiro.

Lopes, E. R., L. M. C. S. Goldfarb, G. A. S. Mendonça, L. A. Marcondes, L. H. Sakamoto, and V. L. C. Silva. 1992. "Cancer and Environment." In M. C. Leal, P. C. Sabroza, R. H. Rodriguez, and P. M. Buss, eds., *Health, Environment and Development: An Interdisciplinary Analysis* (in Portuguese), vol. 2: 197–249. Rio de Janeiro: HUCITEC–ABRASCO.

MDIC/SECEX (Ministry of Development, Industry, and Commerce/Secretary of Foreign Affairs). 2001. *Statistics Annual Report 2001* (in Portuguese). Brasília: MDIC.

MDIC/SRF (Ministry of Development, Industry, and Commerce/Federal Income Bureau). 2000. "Informal Market 1992 to 2000" (in Portuguese). MDIC, Brasília.

Ministry of Health. 1999a. "Mortality Information System" (in Portuguese). Available at <http://www.tabnet.datasus.gov.br/cgi/deftohtm.exe?sim/cnv/obtuf.def>; cited December 1999.

———. 1999b. "Economic Actions for Tobacco Control in Brazil: Reducing Smuggling." In *Data and Facts 1999* (in Portuguese). Rio de Janeiro: Ministry of Health/INCA.

———. 2000a. "Concerning the National Program to Reinforce Family-Based Agriculture and the Tobacco Industry" (in Portuguese). Internal document. Ministry of Health/INCA, Rio de Janeiro.

———. 2000b. "Results of the `Smoke-Free National Cancer Institute' Pilot Project" (in Portuguese). Preliminary analysis. Rio de Janeiro.

Ministry of Health and ASCOM (Social Communication Area). 2000. "Tobacco Control 2000: Impact of Media Campaigns. Analysis Report on the Films *Trafficker* and *Journalist*" (in Portuguese). Ministry of Health, Brasília.

Ministry of Health and IBGE (Brazilian Institute of Geography and Statistics). 1989. "Household Survey on Nutrition and Health" (in Portuguese). IBGE, Rio de Janeiro.

Ministry of Health, INCA (National Cancer Institute), and CONPREV (Tobacco Control, Cancer Prevention, and Surveillance National Coordination). 2001a. *Consensus on Treatment of Tobacco Users* (in Portuguese). Rio de Janeiro: Ministry of Health/INCA.

———. 2001b. "Data Bank/Decentralization Division" (in Portuguese). Ministry of Health/INCA, Rio de Janeiro.

———. 2001c. "Data Bank/School Sector" (in Portuguese). Ministry of Health/INCA, Rio de Janeiro.

———. 2001d. "Data Bank/ Legislation and Economics Sector" (in Portuguese). Ministry of Health/INCA, Rio de Janeiro.

———. 2001e. "Actions on Legislation and Economics." In *Data and Facts 2001* (in Portuguese). Rio de Janeiro: Ministry of Health/INCA.

———. 2001f. "Framework Convention on Tobacco Control (FCTC)." In *Data and Facts 2001* (in Portuguese). Rio de Janeiro: Ministry of Health/INCA.

Ministry of Health, NCTU (National Commission on Tobacco Use), INCA (National Cancer Institute), and CONPREV (Tobacco Control, Cancer Prevention, and Surveillance National Coordination). 2001. "Report on the NCTU's 12th Meeting on Tobacco Use" (in Portuguese). Internal document. Ministry of Health, Rio de Janeiro.

Nielsen Institute. 1996. "Publicity Investment." In *Getúlio Vargas Foundation Report* (in Portuguese). Rio de Janeiro: Getúlio Vargas Foundation.

Otta, L. A. 2001. "Cigarettes Become a Controversial Issue at Mercosur" (in Portuguese). *O Estado São Paulo*, December 27, Economics section, p. 4.

PAHO (Pan American Health Organization). 1992. *Tobacco or Health: Status in the Americas. A Report of the Pan American Health Organization.* Washington, D.C.

Perez, M. D. C. 1990. "Erosion of Agricultural Practices at Cuenca of Pardinho River" (in Portuguese). Ph.D. dissertation. Rio Grande do Sul University, Zaragoza, Brazil.

Quesada, F., and others. 1989. "Annual Needs of Wood as Fuel in Agriculture and Peccary Production on Small Properties in a Gaúcho Municipality" (in Portuguese). *Rural Social Economics* 25 (1): 53–59.

RITC (Research for International Tobacco Control). 1998. "Tobacco Control Research Priorities for Latin America and the Caribbean: The Rio de Janeiro Report." Ottawa.

Rosemberg, J. 1987. *Tabagismo, Sério Problema de Saúde Pública [Tobacco Use: A Public Health Issue]*, 2d ed. São Paulo: ALMED Editora e Livraria Ltda.

Saffer, H. 2000. "Tobacco Advertising and Promotion." In P. Jha and F. Chaloupka, eds., *Tobacco Control in Developing Countries.* New York: Oxford University Press for the World Bank and the World Health Organization.

Silva, V. L. C. 1987. "Smoking Modification Behavior: An Approach to Teenagers in the Brazilian Anti-Smoking Program." In *Annals of 6th World Conference on Smoking or Health, Tokyo, Japan.* Amsterdam: Elsevier Science.

———. 1999. "Study on the Impact of Tobacco Use on Death by Heart Attack among Women Aged between 35 and 59 Years in Rio de Janeiro" (in Portuguese). Ph.D. dissertation. National Public Health School, Oswaldo Cruz Foundation (FIOCRUZ), Rio de Janeiro.

Silva, V. L. C., T. M. Cavalcante, T. P. Feitosa, and L. M. C. S. Goldfarb, eds. 1998a. *Practical Guidelines for Implementing a Tobacco Control Program* (in Portuguese). Rio de Janerio: Ministry of Health/INCA.

Silva, V. L. C., L. M. C. S. Goldfarb, T. M. Cavalcante, T. P. Feitosa, and R. H. S. Mereilles. 1998b. "Talking about Tobacco Use" (in Portuguese). 3d ed. Ministry of Health/INCA, Rio de Janeiro.

Silva, V. L. C., L. M. C. S. Goldfarb, M. Moraes, and S. R. B. Turci, eds. 1999. *Brazilian Cigarettes: Analysis and Proposals to Reduce Consumption* (in Portuguese). Rio de Janeiro: INCA/CONPREV.

Souza Cruz. 1999a. *The Tobacco Grower* (in Portuguese), no. 102. Rio de Janeiro.

———. 1999b. "Annual Report 1999" (in Portuguese). Rio de Janeiro.

———. 2001. "Annual Report 2001" (in Portuguese). Available at <http://www.souzacruz.com.br/sc-relatorio/port/anual/anual.htm>; cited November 10, 2001.

Sunley, E., A. Yurekli, and F. Chaloupka. 2000. "The Design, Administration, and Potential Revenue of Tobacco Excises." In P. Jha and F. Chaloupka, eds., *Tobacco Control In Developing Countries.* New York: Oxford University Press for the World Bank and the World Health Organization.

Sweanor, D. T. 1992. "Canada's Tobacco Tax Policies: Successes and Challenges." Non-Smokers' Rights Association, Toronto.

Tobacco Free Kids. 2001. "Ventilation Technology Does Not Protect People From Secondhand Tobacco Smoke." Factsheet, April 10, 2001. National Center for Tobacco-Free Kids, Washington, D.C. Available at <http://www.tobaccofreekids.org/research/factsheets/pdf/0145.pdf>; accessed January 10, 2003.

Townsend, J., P. Roderick, and J. Cooper. 1994. "Cigarette Smoking According to Socioeconomic Group, Sex, and Age: Effects of Price, Income, and Health Policy." *British Medical Journal* 309: 923–27.

USDHHS (United States Department of Health and Human Services). 1992. "Smoking and Health in the Americas: A 1992 Report of the Surgeon General, in Collaboration with the Pan American Health Organization." Publication CDC 92-8419. USDHHS/Pan American Health Organization, Atlanta, Ga.

———. 1994. "The Health Consequences of Tobacco Use by Young People." In *Preventing Tobacco Use among Young People. A Report of the Surgeon General.* Atlanta, Ga.

WHO (World Health Organization). 1998. "Growing up without Tobacco: Guidelines to the World No Tobacco Day." Geneva.

World Bank. 1999. *Curbing the Epidemic: Governments and the Economics of Tobacco Control.* Development in Practice series. Washington, D.C.

4

Legislation and Applied Economics in the Pursuit of Public Health: Canada

David Sweanor and Ken Kyle

Over the past 20 years, Canada has accomplished a great deal in tobacco control and has much to be pleased about. Part of the success is the result of particularly effective campaigns led by health advocates, both inside and outside the government, and supported by a large number of important organizations. Also important were comprehensive tobacco control strategies at all levels of government, including prevention, protection, and cessation initiatives, as well as bold action by many politicians. The achievements are impressive:

- Coordinated efforts in the 1980s to increase taxes and so reduce the affordability of tobacco products have contributed to significant declines in smoking: in 1965, 50 percent of Canadians age 15 and older smoked, but by 2001 the rate had dropped to 22 percent.
- There is extensive protection from secondhand smoke in workplaces, in public areas, and even in restaurants and bars in some of the larger cities. Canada was the first country to end smoking on international commercial passenger flights, and Canadians played a key role in international efforts to remove secondhand smoke from air travel.
- Efforts to inform consumers about the risks of smoking have led to groundbreaking changes in package labeling, including pictorial warnings covering half of the surface area of cigarette packages.
- Canada has forced the disclosure of additives and many of the toxins in tobacco smoke and has enacted legislation to require changes in tobacco product design.
- The impact of the decline in smoking prevalence is beginning to show up in lung cancer rates among Canadian males age 20 and older. Since 2000, the number of new cases has fallen by 100 per year, from 12,200 in 2000 to 12,000 in 2002 (Canadian Cancer Society 2002).

It is generally believed that Canada has achieved as much as it has because of particularly favorable circumstances that do not exist in other countries. There is, however, little basis for this assumption. Canada battled the same obstacles—low priority for disease prevention, meager tobacco control resources, and general lack of interest in tobacco issues by government and nongovernmental organizations (NGOs)—as faced by most other countries. While the accomplishments are to be applauded, it must be recognized that the success of the tobacco control campaign is also partly explained by the state of affairs 20 years ago: things were so bad then that significant improvements were not hard to achieve. And Canada still has much to work on.

- Tobacco death rates remain very high, and with a rising population, the total number of smokers is about the same as when the tobacco epidemic was first identified.
- Extremely high smoking rates are still found among many segments of Canadian society, especially Aboriginal people.
- Too little attention is given to helping smokers quit or otherwise reduce their risks.
- Many of the individuals and organizations with mandates to reduce disease are still playing only minor roles in the efforts to enact healthy public policies on tobacco control.
- Canada still produces more tobacco per capita than the United States.

With its mixed picture, the Canadian experience provides important lessons, both for those in Canada who are directly involved and for those deciding what to do—and what not to do—in other countries.

A Generation Gap: Before Tobacco Control

There are many reasons for Canada's failure to make major tobacco control inroads prior to the 1980s. Perhaps the most significant was that the public health community never managed to institute policies that would have influenced attitudes about smoking and tobacco use. For their part, the tobacco companies were adept at fostering strong relations with federal and provincial governments and effectively forestalling any measures that could have reduced sales.

Among the obstacles in the way of tobacco control was the increasing affordability of cigarettes. When adjusted for inflation, the real price of cigarettes decreased from the end of World War II until 1982. During those years the economy expanded rapidly and personal incomes rose, making tobacco increasingly affordable. The impact was obvious in the numbers. At the beginning of the 1980s, Canada's per capita consumption of tobacco was among the highest of any country on the planet. Canada also had the dubious distinction of having the highest per capita consumption among OECD (Organisation for Economic Co-operation and Development) countries. Smoking among teenagers age 15–19 was extraordinarily high; in 1979, 46 percent of this group reported being smokers, and 42 percent of them already smoked daily (Health Canada 1991).

There were no legislated restrictions on tobacco advertising and no mandated warning on tobacco packages until 1989. The only "controls" on advertising and labeling were in a voluntary code of conduct that the tobacco industry constantly violated (NSRA 1986).

The tobacco companies appeared to recognize early on that their continued well-being in the face of an avalanche of damning scientific evidence was dependent on ensuring that politicians did not move decisively to curb tobacco consumption. Unlike the health groups, which at that time were generally absent from political discussions, the tobacco industry made itself heard. It had the ear of government and did its best to control the levers of power.

Given that the Canadian tobacco companies have long been owned or controlled by large international companies, this tactic should have come as no surprise. The companies appear to have realized decades ago that if science is not your friend, you had better be sure that governments are. But the success of this strategy in Canada seemed to exceed even its legendary accomplishments elsewhere in the world. When, for instance, the U.S. surgeon general released the landmark 1964 report on smoking and health, which said unequivocally that smoking was the cause of an epidemic of death and disease, the tobacco companies expressed little concern. Even as Judy LaMarsh, then minister of national health and welfare, stood in the House of Commons asserting that the government would take serious action to confront the problem, the Canadian subsidiary of Rothmans made it clear in its annual report that it saw no reason for concern (Rothmans 1964). The fact that a former prime minister of the country, and the former leader of the party then in power, was chairman of the board of Rothmans in Canada at the time may have influenced this stance.

But the tobacco companies did not reach their position of effective protection from political action against their industry by having just one former prime minister in a position of influence. Several former cabinet ministers and senior government advisers have taken jobs with tobacco companies. (Indeed, just recently three senators were simultaneously sitting in Parliament and on tobacco company boards of directors.) Other "political kingpins in waiting" were appointed to tobacco company positions, and tobacco manufacturers were in politically significant areas such as Montréal and Québec City. Tobacco farmers in Canada were also a powerful political force, using their own government-supported research and their influence on export and marketing boards.

The 1980s: A Decade of Change

A combination of circumstances in the early 1980s fundamentally changed the face of tobacco control in Canada. In hindsight, this change might look revolutionary, particularly when compared with the inaction of earlier years, but in fact it was a rather slow and sometimes painful evolutionary process.

A Lesson in Applied Economics

Relatively high inflation in the 1970s caused both the federal and the provincial governments to guard against the erosion of their revenue base by increasing taxes. Both levels of government indexed some taxes to the retail price of specific products, including cigarettes. Each tax increase by one level of government stimulated an increase by the other level. A hike in prices by tobacco companies accelerated this ratcheting.

As a result, after 1981 tobacco prices began increasing in real terms for the first time in 30 years. Then something interesting happened: total cigarette sales starting falling for the first time in 30 years. Canadian health advocates got an unexpected lesson in the principles of price elasticity, and they used this information in the political battle surrounding taxation. (See "The Power of Taxation," on page 87.)

Mounting Evidence and Interest

The mounting scientific evidence of the harm caused by tobacco use solidified the interest and support of many individuals whose "time had come." These included tobacco control advocates who had honed their skills in campaigns in some of the larger cities, fighting for smoke-free public spaces and bans on tobacco advertising on public transportation. They included reporters who were becoming interested in tobacco issues and advocates who were learning by trial and error (particularly in Toronto) how to work with the print and electronic media. And they even included public servants in the federal health department who, because of personal interest, developed their knowledge about tobacco and became serious about reducing the death and disease that result from tobacco use.

Many of these people had come of age during a time of social activism and had witnessed individuals successfully working together to protest wars, influence environmental policy, push for civil rights, and accomplish other social goals. As tobacco products became recognized as major killers, it was not surprising that many of these people were inspired to take on the cause of tobacco control as another area of social activism.

Institutional Response and Coalition Building

By far the single most important development in the movement for tobacco control in Canada was the founding of the Non-Smokers' Rights Association (NSRA) in Toronto in 1974 by a small group of social activists. From the beginning, the NSRA combined concern for the rights of non-smokers with an interest in pushing for policy changes that would reduce the overall death toll from tobacco use.

Garfield Mahood was hired as the association's first executive director. He had already developed social activist skills as head of an environmental law association and had been successful in working on other social issues. His success in achieving policy breakthroughs attracted the attention of others who shared the view that political activism could save lives. One of them was a young lawyer, David Sweanor, who by 1983 was working full-time alongside Mahood and trying hard to match his feverish intensity.

Around this time, a chance incident provided the catalyst for the formation of a tobacco control lobby. In 1985 the federal minister of agriculture proposed the creation of a national Flue-Cured Tobacco Marketing Agency to promote the sale of Canadian tobacco at home and abroad. A number of health groups decided to make presentations to the government to oppose this initiative. Some individuals from these organizations found themselves waiting in the same room for the presentations to begin, and it occurred to them that there might be advantages to cooperation. So, despite being told by senior government officials and members of the media that there was no chance of derailing the marketing board concept, they increased the pressure through media advocacy and other measures that made a "done deal" look badly in need of serious reexamination. Soon, the tobacco industry itself became splintered on the issues involved, and the idea of a marketing board fell apart. A lesson learned: seemingly irresistible forces within the tobacco industry could be successfully challenged by effective advocacy.

A partnership soon developed between this fast-response advocacy group and the biggest, most prestigious voluntary health charity in the country, the Canadian Cancer Society (CCS). The main function of the CCS up to this point had been to raise funds for medical research through a massive door-to-door campaign held every April. The organization also had a long history of conducting health promotion programs, providing support to cancer patients, and disseminating information on cancer. But by 1986 the CCS decided that it needed to become more involved in advocacy. Ken Kyle was hired as director of public issues, and he was instrumental in building a coalition with the NSRA to work on tobacco control.

With a few key committed people taking hold of the political levers and feeding off each other's knowledge and enthusiasm, it did not take long for support for the coalition to grow. After a few years other health groups became involved: first, the Heart and Stroke Foundation of Canada and, to a lesser extent, the Canadian Lung Association and the Canadian Medical Association. The Canadian Council on Smoking and Health (CCSH, now the Canadian Council for Tobacco), which was initially run by staff of the three health charities, was part of the coalition from the start. Other civil society groups such as the United Church of Canada, labor unions, and women's groups played a smaller but supportive role.

Forging Links between Research and Advocacy

By the early 1980s a strong body of evidence concerning the impact of tobacco product pricing on consumption and the danger of secondhand smoke had been developed, and there was clear recognition of the need for serious governmental action in reaction to this evidence and of the effect that advocacy could have in achieving public health objectives. More important, the information from researchers was finding its way to government officials and to health advocates. Academics, often frustrated because research that could save lives was not readily adopted and embodied in government policy, took note of the actions of advocates and sought them out to present useful information. Some of the key data on advertising, taxation, and secondhand smoke made its way to advocates in this fashion. Other researchers and medical specialists, inspired by the publicity garnered by the advocates' activities, were increasingly receptive to their requests for expert assistance. Advocacy groups such as the NSRA quickly learned that success in public health battles brought more opportunities for progress, including the impetus to build alliances.

Working for Policy Change: An Overview

Successful advocates learn to take advantage of opportunities as they arise and to respond quickly and creatively. But long-term strategies are important too. As the tobacco control lobby moved toward working at senior levels of government in pursuit of significant policy change and law reform, the "rapid response" approach had to be effectively integrated with long-term efforts, and the strategy shifted from short-term battles toward a long-term campaign. Health advocates learned to set objectives and use their relative advantages of information, science, energy, quickness, and dedication to achieve them.

Of the many policy initiatives on tobacco control proposed over the past 20 years in Canada (see the Appendix to this chapter), those discussed in this section best illustrate successful strategies for policy change on this important issue. These examples may be helpful to others seeking information and inspiration for policy change.

The Advertising Tug-of-War

At the time the NSRA was formed, the tobacco industry faced no advertising restrictions in Canada. Advertisements showed up everywhere and were accepted as part of the landscape. The NSRA recognized that any efforts it or other groups made to help smokers quit were sure to be swamped by massive advertising designed to entice new recruits. As Mahood commented in media interviews at the time, "It is like trying to bail a boat while someone else drills a hole in its bottom."

The NSRA therefore began by producing background information on the detrimental effects of tobacco advertising and put together comprehensive arguments for restricting or eliminating tobacco advertisements. In those early days the NSRA did not have the organization or resources to lobby effectively for a nationally legislated end to tobacco advertising, so it set its sights on a smaller target. It launched a campaign to have tobacco advertising removed from the popular Toronto Transit Commission (TTC), the busiest transit system in Canada, which carried over 400 million passengers a year on its subways, streetcars, and buses—and exposed them to continuous enticements to smoke cigarettes. The tobacco industry fought hard against the effort to limit its advertising in the TTC and was supported by advertising agencies, billboard companies, and some newspapers and magazine publishers, all of which benefited financially from the advertising.

In 1979, after a two-year battle supported by a loose coalition of other health groups and backed by Emerson Foote, a living legend in the advertising business, the transit authority agreed to drop the advertisements. Those with a vested interest in tobacco advertising were not pleased to have been beaten.

A battle had been won, and a war began. What had been learned was that the tobacco industry seemed to have a hard time with constantly moving targets. The tobacco control health lobby built on this lesson with a strategy of using numerous individual efforts to move creatively and methodically toward the long-term goal of ending tobacco product promotion. Much of the initial leadership in the campaign for the advertising ban came from Mahood and Sweanor of the NSRA, but there was also a great deal of support from Victor Lachance of the Canadian Council on Smoking and Health and Ken Kyle, whose CCS office in downtown Ottawa became known as the "war room." Pro–public health civil servants like Neil Collishaw also began to have a more receptive audience for the work being done inside the government on tobacco control. As the core group of strategists grew, and as other health groups gradually began to focus on tobacco issues, the realm of what might be achievable also expanded.

As the campaign moved forward, no one was ever quite sure what would happen next. But the next step came suddenly. In 1983 the Canadian subsidiary of the RJR-Macdonald tobacco company became the sponsor of the Canadian Ski Association, allowing the firm to associate cigarettes and smoking with skiers who were national heroes. Many of the skiers and the team physicians were appalled. They opposed the decision of their governing body and decided to fight the sponsorship. What could have been a coup for the tobacco industry became a rallying point for the health lobby. Health and medical groups that had long paid lip service to public health without getting involved in tobacco control were forced to take positions as the debate heated up. The tobacco promotional contracts with the ski association were leaked, and protests were held. Eventually, the skiers themselves stole the show by refusing to accept trophies associated with cigarettes, and they publicly denounced the tobacco company sponsorship. All of this publicity assisted the federal minister of health, who was under pressure on other tobacco issues, to cut government subsidies for sporting bodies that accepted funding from the tobacco industry.

The industry countered any call for legislation by trumpeting both its own voluntary code on advertising and the voluntary self-regulation of the advertising industry. Before legislation could reasonably be expected, the health groups had to prove that these existing measures were ineffective.

Efforts by a member of the public helped the cause. Ed Flis, a Canadian citizen, had written several letters to the tobacco companies during the 1970s in an effort to force the industry to define what it actually meant by the statements in its code of conduct. This was a spontaneous action by a citizen who was simply interested in doing something about tobacco's toll on society. Flis turned the responses over to the NSRA, and suddenly the health lobby had operational definitions of the code—for example, what the tobacco industry meant by terms such as "immediate vicinity" in reference to the rule about keeping tobacco advertisements away from schools.

Armed with this evidence, the health lobby was able to show that the voluntary codes were totally ineffective. In 1984 the NSRA released a list of 250 billboards with tobacco advertisements that were within the proscribed distance from schools. Complaints were also filed with the self-regulatory body of the advertising industry. The responses to those complaints suggested an unwillingness to remove a single tobacco ad. Even when the complaints were backed by the expert opinions of epidemiologists, linguists, and lawyers, which left no doubt that the voluntary code had been violated, the initial reaction was to amend the code to allow the complained-of practice. In 1986 the NSRA prepared a major report, *A Catalogue of Deception*, that documented ongoing violations of virtually every rule in the voluntary code. Some of them were blatant. For example, according to Rule 7, advertising was to be addressed only to adults over 18, but Imperial Tobacco paid to have its brand name and logo on the centerfold map of the guidebook to Toronto's "Canada's Wonderland," whose roller coasters and other attractions are designed for children under 18. Rule 1 stated that there would be no advertising or promotion of sponsorships of sports or other popular events through the use of brand names, corporate names, or logos on radio or television, but tobacco logos and brands were constantly seen on televised coverage of sports and other events sponsored by the tobacco industry.

In 1986 Health Minister Jake Epp acknowledged that self-regulation of tobacco advertising was ineffective. What really pushed the government into legislative action, however, was a private member's bill sponsored by Lynn McDonald, a member of Parliament from an opposition party and a fierce opponent of smoking. (Private members' bills are sponsored by individual members of Parliament, not by the government, and rarely pass into law.)

McDonald's bill, introduced in the House of Commons in October 1986, proposed regulating smoking in federally regulated workplaces and placing tobacco under the Hazardous Products Act. This would mean that tobacco advertising would be prohibited unless exempted by specific provisions. Health groups pressured members of Parliament from all parties to support the bill. Eventually, the government decided to draft its own bill banning tobacco advertising, and in 1987 Minister Epp introduced such legislation. The resulting Tobacco Products Control Act was enacted in 1988 and came into force on January 1, 1989. McDonald's bill, entitled the Non-Smokers Health Act, also passed, without the section on advertising but with the sections on smoking in public space. (See "Achieving Smoke-Free Space," on page 84.)

The goal of moving the government into action had been met, but the war was just heating up. The tobacco industry poured massive sums of money into efforts to derail the legislation. It hired additional lobbyists, including Bill Neville, who was very close to the prime minister and was well connected with virtually the entire federal cabinet. Neville was considered the most powerful lobbyist in the country and was purportedly paid more than any lobbyist in Canada had ever received.

Neville's power was undermined by the health groups, which delighted in pointing out his personal connections—this at a time when there was great public interest in eliminating personal influence that subverted due process in government. In what many considered to be a master stroke of the campaign, the health lobby ran a full-page advertisement in the national newspaper, the *Globe and Mail,* showing a picture of the prime minister next to a picture of Neville and accompanied by an appeal to put the interests of Canadian children ahead of the interests of the tobacco companies. The health lobby also exposed some tobacco industry deceptions, most notably when it showed that an influx of letters to members of Parliament, designed to look like public opposition to the law, actually consisted of letters composed and printed by the tobacco lobby.

Meanwhile, advocates worked hard to build public support for an advertising ban through news conferences, paid newspaper advertisements, pamphlets, and the publication of favorable polling results. The CCS organized a campaign to send 35,000 black-bordered postcards (one for every tobacco-related death that year) to members of Parliament. The Canadian Medical Association asked its members to vote against any member of Parliament who did not support the bill. An equally important part of the lobby was the "inside" strategy, whereby health groups worked with the minister of health and his advisers, officials of the health department, and members of Parliament sitting on the legislative committee reviewing the proposed law.

The tobacco industry responded to the passage of the Tobacco Products Control Act with continual efforts to undermine the impact of the regulations. And it launched a successful court challenge: in 1995 the Supreme Court of Canada ruled that a total ban on tobacco advertising was unconstitutional, effectively invalidating important provisions of the act.

Health groups reacted immediately to this setback by launching a campaign for new legislation controlling tobacco advertising and promotion. In November 1996 the health minister, David Dingwall, introduced a new bill, the Tobacco Act, which sought to outlaw most existing tobacco advertising but allowed limited advertising in publications with a mostly adult readership, through direct mail, and in places where young people are prohibited, such as bars. It also incorporated the provisions of the Tobacco Sales to Young Persons Act, which had come into force in 1994. That Act raised the minimum age for buying tobacco to age 18, restricted tobacco vending machines to bars and taverns, and set hefty fines for infractions. The new Tobacco Act furthermore provided for the first government-approved product design standards, package labeling that included health messages, regular industry reports to Health Canada on a variety of matters, and restrictions on tobacco sponsorship advertising.

The tobacco control lobby, which became known as the National Campaign for Action on Tobacco, campaigned heavily. Particularly important this time was the existence within major health organizations of professionals who by now had many years of experience in lobbying for tobacco control legislation. Key campaign participants included the NSRA, the CCS, and Physicians for a Smoke-Free Canada. The Heart and Stroke Foundation of

Canada and the Canadian Lung Association lobbied more actively this time. A new and important player was the Coalition québécoise pour le contrôle du tabac (Québec Coalition for Tobacco Control).

Despite growing support for tobacco control, the campaign still had weaknesses, including a lack of initiative by some health groups, poor coordination within the whole health community, and the usual lack of financial resources (May 1988). The tobacco industry seemed to be always organized and vigorous in its opposition to the campaign, particularly over the issue of tobacco advertising through sponsorship. The industry even established a lobbying group, the Alliance for Sponsorship Freedom, to fight the new law. This group, consisting of organizations receiving tobacco sponsorship money, was funded by the tobacco industry and was run through a public relations firm directed by the industry. The industry also engaged in tough direct lobbying, including extensive media advertising.

Many of the sports and cultural events sponsored by the tobacco industry were held in the province of Québec, and the opposition Bloc Québécois in Parliament did not support the proposed sponsorship restrictions. The minister of health eventually agreed to amendments that delayed the bill by two years. Lobbying activities were then redirected to the Senate, where the bill had still to be approved. With a federal election expected shortly, the industry strategy was to force delays so that the bill would not be debated and passed in Parliament before the election. The bill finally passed the Senate on April 16, 1997, less than two weeks before Parliament was dissolved for the election, but in order to get it through caucus, Health Minister Dingwall had to agree to introduce a new bill after the election to allow tobacco sponsorship of international automobile races.

The new minister of health, Allan Rock, introduced such a bill in June 1998. This Act to Amend the Tobacco Act delayed the implementation date for partial restrictions on tobacco sponsorship from October 1, 2000 to October 1, 2003. Nevertheless, Minister Rock showed an important commitment to tobacco control through a new provision, contained in the bill, to ban all tobacco sponsorship advertising by October 2003. Parliament passed the bill on December 10, 1998.

A Picture Worth a Thousand Words: Product Labeling

Under Canadian law and the laws of many other countries, manufacturers are obligated to warn consumers about the nature and extent of any hazards associated with their products. The warning must be clearly communicated and must not be negated by collateral efforts on the part of manufacturers.

In Canada from 1972 to 1989 the only warning on cigarette packages was one placed voluntarily by the tobacco companies. It appeared in very small type on the side of tobacco packages and read, "Danger to health increases with amount smoked. Avoid inhaling." Health groups had long argued that better information should be provided to consumers, but it was not until the 1980s that a serious campaign for legislated messages was launched.

After some discussion, the tobacco control lobby agreed to press for large pictorial warning messages and for further information on the inside of tobacco packaging. This particular campaign benefited from one of the most effective combinations of NGOs, the Office of the Minister of Health, and federal bureaucrats, working as true partners. It also saw far more use of scientific studies and focus groups than in earlier campaigns.

A major problem was the lack of a clear agreement on standards for "informed consent." The tobacco industry has consistently claimed that smokers understand smoking may be harmful. Health advocates argued that a much more rigorous standard of informed consent with respect to the harm caused by tobacco products was appropriate and that the level of detail of the information provided should be more like that required of the pharmaceutical and automobile industries. The existing warning on cigarette packs conveyed little more than a vague notion of the existence of some risk and did nothing to list the specific risks or to quantify them for smokers.

Tobacco control advocates aimed to ensure by regulation that worthwhile information would be provided by the tobacco companies themselves as a condition for their selling their products. They began by raising awareness of the need for more information. Consumer surveys were conducted, and past surveys from the federal health department were obtained under freedom of information laws. The results were astounding. The surveys revealed that smokers, and young people in the age group most likely to initiate smoking, were unable to name many of the diseases caused by smoking. Most could not even recall that smoking caused heart disease—the single biggest cause of death due to tobacco use (Environics Research Group Ltd. 1990).

Health groups were successful in using results from medical research and public opinion surveys to instigate hard-hitting media advocacy campaigns for legislative reform. Complaints were filed under provincial trade practices legislation accusing tobacco companies of violating provisions of the laws that prohibit "deception by omission"—failure to state material facts, so that consumers are deceived or tend to be deceived. There were also coalition news conferences and newspaper articles about the lack of effective and truthful health messages on cigarette packaging, and comparisons with the countries that did have legislated package warnings.

The Tobacco Products Control Act created a legislative framework for regulating package health warnings. Regulations under the act called for cigarette packages to display prominent warnings in contrasting colors covering 20 percent of each of the main panels of both cigarette packs and cartons. The tobacco industry complied, but barely. Suddenly, the "contrasting colors" turned out to be silver on white, gold on brown, and other combinations that made the warnings hard to read easily. The "main package panel" on cartons was interpreted by the industry as the smallest panel—the ends of the cartons, rather than the sides, obviously contrary to the intent of the act.

The tobacco control coalition turned this short-term setback into a powerful tool for even better package warnings. It exposed to politicians, bureaucrats, and the media the wording of the regulations and the tobacco industry's interpretation of them. Typical responses were anger, laughter, or both. In June 1989 the NSRA released to the public information it had obtained showing how the tobacco industry had succeeded in weakening the warnings during the regulatory process. The industry may have won a temporary delay against better warnings, but it lost credibility. In January 1990 the coalition celebrated success when the minister of health, Perrin Beatty, announced that the regulations would be revised in July 1991 to require eight rotating messages covering the top 25 percent of the front and back of the packages and printed in black and white—not the package colors.

Over the next several months, the issue of the regulations went back and forth. The tobacco control coalition lobbied the new minister of health, Benoit Bouchard, not to implement the new regulations. The NSRA and the Heart and Stroke Foundation of Canada sent pamphlets to the households of the electoral districts of all the members of the cabinet committee that would be deciding on the new (weakened) regulations. A survey by Health Canada found that smokers liked the new proposals for bigger warnings better than the old format. Finally, in 1993 another new minister of health, Mary Collins, pushed the new warnings through the cabinet with an implementation date of September 12, 1994.

After all that, in 1995 the Supreme Court of Canada, as part of its ruling on the Tobacco Products Control Act (see "The Advertising Tug-of-War," on page 77), narrowly decided in favor of the tobacco industry, saying that it was unconstitutional to mandate health warnings unless they were attributed to the government. The tobacco industry's argument was that free speech included the right to silence and that the existence of mandatory but unattributed messages gave the erroneous impression that the tobacco industry was itself giving the warnings.

Despite its victory in court, the tobacco industry was in no position to remove the "unconstitutional" messages. Doing so would have raised serious problems in pending product liability cases and would also have angered legislators. The warnings stayed virtually unchanged for the time being, although the industry made it clear that new legislation would be needed if the warnings were to exist in the future. Within three years, the new Tobacco Act, containing even broader powers to regulate warnings, was passed. In January 1999 Health Minister Rock released a discussion paper that proposed expanding the warnings to the top 60 percent of the front and back of packages and giving additional information, such as cessation tips and reference to a Website, on the inside of packs. In April the coalition researched and then released to the media and politicians mock-ups of the warnings, which helped greatly with political support.

On January 19, 2000, Minister Rock made public 16 pictorial messages that were to appear in rotation on 50 percent of the front and back of packs (see figure 4.1). Some of the pictures were gruesome, but research from both the federal Department of Health and the CCS showed these warnings to be more effective than text-only ones.

The final regulations received unanimous approval (a rarity) by both the House of Commons Committee and the House of Commons and were then approved by the cabinet. The Tobacco Products Information Regulations became law on June 26, 2000.[1]

Reaching the goal of providing better information to smokers is an ongoing battle that has taken a lot of hard work. It has been aided, however, by the ability of Canadian health advocates to use research and advocacy to turn defeats into victories, codified in new government policy and legislation. Things that seem to be obstacles can in fact open up new opportunities. The key is the ability to see the opportunities when others might see only obstacles.

Achieving Smoke-Free Space

Protecting the public from secondhand smoke was always considered an important public health goal, given the acute and chronic health problems resulting from exposure. As with all the other major Canadian efforts on tobacco control, it was possible for advocates to determine a long-term goal and then choose appropriate tactics for short-term efforts aimed at eventually allowing Canadians to be free from secondhand smoke.

By the mid-1970s community-based groups of activists such as the NSRA were involved in efforts to get municipal bylaws that would offer protection from secondhand smoke. To begin with, the goals were seemingly modest:

---

1. Details can be found on Health Canada's Website, <www.hc-sc.gc.ca/english/tobacco.htm>.

Figure 4.1. Examples of Canadian Pictorial Warning Labels for Cigarette Packages

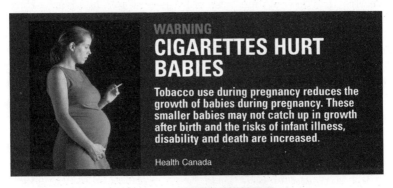

WARNING
CIGARETTES HURT BABIES

Tobacco use during pregnancy reduces the growth of babies during pregnancy. These smaller babies may not catch up in growth after birth and the risks of infant illness, disability and death are increased.

Health Canada

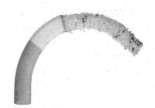

AVERTISSEMENT
LE TABAGISME PEUT VOUS RENDRE IMPUISSANT

La cigarette peut provoquer l'impuissance sexuelle car elle réduit la circulation du sang dans le pénis. Cela peut vous rendre incapable d'avoir une érection.

Santé Canada

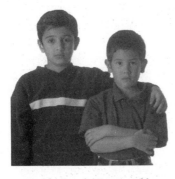

DON'T POISON US

WARNING: Second-hand smoke contains carbon monoxide, ammonia, formaldehyde, benzo[a]pyrene and nitrosamines. These chemicals can harm your children.

Health Canada

Source: Health Canada. Reprinted by permission.

prohibiting smoking in elevators, food stores, and other confined spaces. The groups recognized that the most dramatic efforts, such as pushing for smoking bans in public areas, were the least likely to be effective. Several cities, including Victoria, Vancouver, Edmonton, Toronto, and Ottawa, passed the more limited laws. As the public grew used to them, amendments were gradually introduced to broaden their scope.

Efforts moved to the national level in 1986 when, as described above, Lynn McDonald introduced the Non-Smokers Health Act in the House of Commons. This private member's bill was designed to ensure protection from secondhand smoke in federally regulated workplaces. Although it was given little chance of success, it gathered growing support and managed to dodge various efforts to have it killed.

Much of the credit for the eventual enactment of the bill goes to Cynthia Callard, now executive director of Physicians for a Smoke-Free Canada, who was at the time an assistant to McDonald. She brought to the effort a passion for public health, knowledge of the Canadian parliamentary system, and an ability to get others involved. McDonald's bill provided the catalyst for the government to draft its own bill limiting tobacco advertising, the Tobacco Products Control Act (see "The Advertising Tug-of-War," on page 77). The two bills ended up traveling together through the legislative process. Every effort by the tobacco industry to stop them was countered, and each bill helped the other move forward.

On May 31, 1988, both bills were passed by the House of Commons in an extraordinary vote in which members voted as individuals rather than along party lines. The power of the tobacco lobby and its advocacy groups, and its questionable claims of little harm from secondhand smoke, had been beaten back.

The Non-Smokers' Health Act essentially gave all federally regulated workers (about 10 percent of Canada's workforce) the right to a smoke-free workplace. Flight attendants, passenger train workers, and intercity bus drivers fell under the law and received the right to be free from cigarette smoke. Naturally, implementation was a challenge. Many of the companies involved, including the airlines, claimed that the law would put them out of business. The airlines were particularly effective in obtaining extensions of the deadline due to concerns about competition on international routes.

But the health lobby pressed forward. The flight length for smoke-free aircraft was gradually increased until all flights except those to Asia were covered, and then that exemption was also eliminated. Canada became the first country to have all flights of its airlines smoke-free. As it turned out, not only was there no competitive disadvantage; the airlines found that the clean air policy attracted business from competitors. In only a short time other airlines recognized the advantages of smoke-free travel, and within a few years virtually all the major air carriers were smoke-free.

Airlines were not the only battleground for the implementation of the new law. At one point the government nearly passed a regulation that would have exempted intercity buses from the nonsmoking law. Rather than attack the government plan, the NSRA and the CCS approached the bus companies directly. It was pointed out that other forms of transportation were going smoke-free and that the buses would suffer from a "lower-class" image if they continued to allow smoking. This happened precisely when the industry was trying to move up-market. The result was that the bus companies demanded to be designated smoke-free, proving that allies can often be found when they are creatively sought.

The federal law led the way, but provincial regulations were not far behind, as smoke-free spaces became the norm. Meanwhile, the fight for further protection from secondhand smoke moved to restaurants and bars, previously thought to be off-limits to clean air policies. In many cases this move was voluntary, but to give a consistent level of protection, legislation was needed. As with earlier efforts to clear the air, the first steps were taken at the municipal level. By 2002 most of Canada's largest cities either had smoke-free bars and restaurants or were in the process of making them so. It has been a long journey from the days of fighting to get smoking out of food stores and elevators, but there was never doubt about the eventual achievement of the broader goal.

The Power of Taxation

The affordability of tobacco products has repeatedly proved to be the single biggest factor in determining per capita consumption (World Bank 1999). As with virtually all other products, as prices increase, consumption decreases. Yet, as in other countries, Canadian health advocates were rather slow in turning this fundamental law of economics into a public health tool.

In 1983 it began to be clear that price was a very powerful factor in cigarette sales. As a result of the indexation of taxes, cigarette prices began to show a sustained increase in real terms for the first time in over 30 years. There was an immediate impact: total cigarette sales began to fall—something the country had not previously experienced.

Some very good analyses of the price elasticity of tobacco products had already been done, primarily in the United States and the United Kingdom, and they had been replicated for Canada and disseminated by Neil Collishaw at the federal health department. But although the tax structure in place was a huge benefit to public health, it was under attack by the tobacco industry, as well as alcohol companies, which had been subject to the same escalating taxes. Under pressure from these interests, the federal government set up a committee to review the taxes and recommend changes. The members of the committee came from the tobacco and alcohol industries; not one representative of health groups was invited to attend, nor did any health groups (except for one that sent a single letter) make any submissions to the committee or to the government. The result was that the indexed tax increases were repealed.

But once again, a defeat paved the way for a much greater victory. In 1984 the Progressive Conservative Party was elected to form the government. After an advocacy campaign led by David Sweanor of the NSRA, the new finance minister, Michael Wilson, raised tobacco taxes by a penny a cigarette in 1985. Consumption fell once more, and health advocates began to understand the relationship between prices and consumption. Under the NSRA's leadership, an organized effort began to take shape to press for greatly increased tobacco taxes (NSRA 1992).

Once again, health advocates set a long-range goal and started working on the building blocks necessary to reach it. In the early stages the efforts were relatively simple. Letters and submissions were sent to governments, presenting both the health justification for tobacco tax increases and the sales and revenue implications, using the best available estimates of price elasticity for cigarettes. In some cases meetings were held with civil servants and political advisers involved in crafting budgets. These efforts began to show results. Government officials were often very pleased to have health advocates talk about tobacco taxes, occasionally mentioning how for years they had been lobbied by the tobacco industry and had always wanted to get the perspective of "the other side."

But significant obstacles stood in the way of imposing higher tobacco taxes. Perhaps the biggest was that posed by Ontario. The province was, after North Carolina and Kentucky, the largest grower of tobacco in North America, and its tobacco taxes were among the lowest of any province. A new provincial government had just been elected, and the minister of finance was a long-serving politician from the "tobacco belt." He was on record as opposing any tobacco tax increase because of the impact on tobacco farmers, and one of the first acts of his government was to rescind a pending tobacco tax hike. Ontario represented well over 35 percent of the nation's population, and its low tobacco prices acted as a ceiling that kept neighboring provinces' taxes lower. It was critical that the "Ontario obstacle" be removed.

To that end, the NSRA conducted an analysis of the impact of rescinding the previously announced tobacco tax increase. Particular attention was paid to tobacco growers. Tobacco leaf is an exceedingly tiny part of the price of manufactured cigarettes—a fact often overlooked when concern for tobacco farmers is used as a justification for not increasing taxes. In late October 1985 the NSRA put together figures showing that the government was forgoing revenues of over 130 million Canadian dollars (CA$), equivalent to US$95 million, in order to maintain higher sales that amounted to the average production of only a dozen farms (Sweanor 1985).

On November 1, 1985, the NSRA held a press conference at the Ontario Legislature denouncing the tax decision as both a blow to public health and possibly the least cost-effective farm support scheme that any government had ever devised. The media were not used to hearing economic arguments from health advocates. Some of the reporters called government finance officials for verification and were told that the NSRA analysis was correct. The next day, both the analysis and a statement by a senior civil servant agreeing with it were published in the *Globe and Mail*.

Momentum was building. Soon there was a coalition, including the NSRA and health charities, that supported significant tobacco tax increases in Ontario and recommended that some of the revenue raised be directed to helping displaced tobacco farmers. Despite his early pro-tobacco leanings, which had earned him the moniker "Tobacco Bob," the finance minister delivered the two biggest tobacco tax increases in Ontario's history during his five years in office. He also funded realistic efforts to help tobacco growers diversify.

While this was going on in Ontario, complementary actions were occurring in all of the other provinces and at the federal level. Ongoing meetings with government officials, political advisers, and cabinet ministers were held. Tobacco industry submissions were obtained (usually under freedom of information laws) and critiqued. The CCS, the Canadian Medical Association, and the Canadian Council on Smoking and Health were making effective use of their staffs and volunteers in various efforts across the country to bring forward tax submissions and meet with decisionmakers. The submissions were primarily produced by the NSRA, which had developed expertise in this area. By the late 1980s provincial governments were calling the NSRA for information on tobacco taxes and for recommendations on how big the tax increases should be.

The federal government increased its tobacco taxes by more than 6 cents a cigarette between 1985 and 1991 as the "tobacco tax project" geared up, and provincial governments roughly matched this level of increase. As expected, consumption fell dramatically. According to Health Canada and Statistics Canada figures, reported domestic sales dropped by 40 percent between 1982 and 1992. Health Canada prevalence surveys also showed that teenagers, who had long been shown to be price-sensitive, achieved a per capita decline of 60 percent. Whereas the 1979 survey showed that 42 percent of 15- to 19-year-olds were daily smokers, by 1991 only 16 percent were (Statistics Canada n.d.).

In response to the tax increases, the tobacco industry fought back. This time, it focused on the issue of cigarette smuggling. At the time, cigarette prices in the United States were less than half those in Canada. The tobacco industry argued that if the price differential remained, a smuggling problem would soon develop.

There was little evidence in the late 1980s and early 1990s to back up this industry position. Canadians were smoking different brands and different tobacco blends than Americans, and sales of U.S. brands in Canada (both legal and otherwise) were declining. But in the early 1990s "exports" of Canadian cigarettes to the United States surged. At the same time, there seemed to be an increase in smuggled cigarettes coming into Canada. Interestingly, these smuggled cigarettes were Canadian blends and Canadian brands—the very ones that were being "exported" in the first place.

The tobacco companies and their allies meanwhile claimed that smuggling was a huge threat to the country and urged governments to lower tobacco taxes as the only way to deal with the scourge. Cigarette retailers joined in the effort to secure a tax rollback in hopes of reclaiming lost sales. In February 1994 the new Liberal government responded by drastically reducing tobacco taxes. As figures 4.2 and 4.3 suggest, there was some increase in consumption, especially among young Canadians. The tax rollbacks lost much of the ground that had been gained since 1982 and poisoned relations between tobacco control advocates and government officials for several years.

The smuggling problem went away as if someone had suddenly turned off a tap (NSRA 1994). There was considerable controversy about the actual level of smuggling and hence of total consumption. Many people argued that the high taxes had "caused" smuggling. They certainly provided an incentive to smuggle, but seeing them as the "cause" of smuggling is like describing an iceberg as a chunk of ice sticking up from the ocean—true as far as it goes, but not the full story at all. The key question is where the smuggled cigarettes were coming from—who was supplying the illegal market? Most of the smuggled cigarettes were manufactured in Canada and exported to the United States, where there was little demand for Canadian brands. Did the exporters think their cigarettes would stay in the United States, or did they know that they would be smuggled back into Canada? Eventually, one of the tobacco companies entered a guilty plea in a U.S. court, admitting to having knowingly played a role in the smuggling. A criminal investigation was instituted in Canada.

Recently, taxes have again been on the increase and now exceed early 1994 levels in all provinces. With every increase, though, consumption declines. These tax and consumption trends continue to be monitored by the NSRA, the CCS, and Physicians for a Smoke-Free Canada.

Working through the Courts for Policy Change

Lawsuits have been used effectively in Canada in the long-term campaign for tobacco control. Using the court system to effect policy change is a

Figure 4.2. Cigarette Consumption and Real Cigarette Prices, Canada, 1949–98

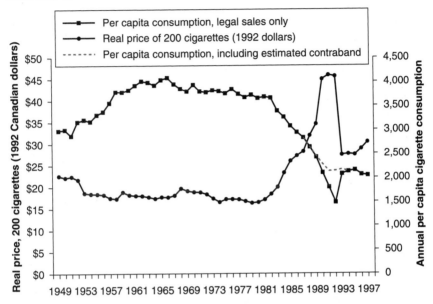

Note: Real prices are calculated from the consumer price index. In high-smuggling years the effective price was lower because smuggled cigarettes evade taxes and are sold at prices below the retail prices of legally sold cigarettes. Consumption data include the highest credible estimate of contraband sales. Cigarettes include fine-cut tobacco equivalents (1 g).

Source: NSRA data.

lengthy process and is sometimes unpredictable, but the ultimate positive results can be large and durable.

In a few provinces laws have been used to bring the tobacco industry to court. For example, in 1997 the legislature of British Columbia passed the Tobacco Damages Recovery Act to assist the provincial government in a lawsuit to recover from the industry costs related to provision of publicly funded hospital and physician services. (The act's title was later changed to the Tobacco Damages and Health Care Costs Recovery Act.) The provincial government then filed an action in the British Columbia Supreme Court against the tobacco industry. The industry challenged the constitutionality of the legislation, and in February 2000 the court ruled the act invalid but upheld some of its major principles. The legislature again amended the act, and the government has launched a new lawsuit.

Ontario passed similar legislation in 1999: the Ministry of Health and Long-Term Care Statute Law Amendment Act. In March 2000 the provincial

Figure 4.3. Smoking Prevalence among Teenagers Age 15–19, Regular Smokers, Canada, 1977–94

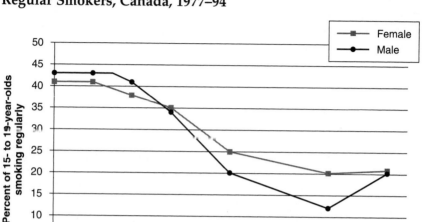

Source: NSRA, using Statistics Canada catalogues 91-002, 91-512, and 91-213; labor force survey data from Statistics Canada (1991); and "Survey on Canada," cycle 3, 1994.

government filed a lawsuit against the industry in U.S. Federal Court under the Racketeer Influenced and Corrupt Organizations (RICO) Act, but in August 2000 the case was dismissed on the grounds that the provincial government could not sue in a U.S. court. The provincial government is planning an appeal.

Newfoundland has also recently passed a Tobacco Health Care Costs Recovery Act, originally introduced in December 2000.

Lessons Learned

There were, of course, many other battles on other aspects of tobacco control, and there was much more to each of the examples cited above than can be adequately conveyed in a few pages. Yet the same lessons seem to shine through. A small group of dedicated people truly can—and did— change the world. They had to set long-term goals and to work realistically toward achieving them. They had to look for allies in the government and beyond, to work with the media, and to take advantage of opportunities as they arose. They had to use research—both their own and from other organizations—to obtain the information they needed in good time and provide it to decisionmakers and the public. They had to be creative, and, for long-term success, they had to have enough sense of camaraderie and accomplishment to want to stay in the fight.

Some other general lessons learned along the way may inform others in their own efforts.

Dealing with an Oligopoly

The tobacco industry in Canada, as in so many other countries, is composed of a very small number of companies that control roughly 99 percent of the market. A single company, Imperial Tobacco Ltd., holds roughly two-thirds of the entire market. Profit margins have traditionally been huge. This gives the tobacco industry a great interest in opposing measures that threaten to curtail the market plus virtually unlimited financial resources for backing its opposition to measures not to its liking. In more competitive markets, the expenditure of millions of dollars on lawyers to fight government legislation would lower a company's profits and make it uncompetitive in the long run. But in the case of the oligopolistic cigarette market, as long as the companies are all in it together, the cost of litigation, lobbyists, "science" to order, and so on is not a problem. The companies can raise prices to cover the costs and continue to realize enormous profits.

Globally, the industry is consolidating rather than becoming more competitive. Countries with competition laws that have been used to combat concentrations or lack of price competition in other industries have not so far opposed consolidation of cigarette companies or tried to curb the power of the cigarette cartels. The companies remain economically powerful and use their resources to build political influence, creating a formidable barrier to tobacco control policy. This makes transparency and public debate on proposed legislation extremely important.

Understanding the Nature of Effective Legislation

Canadian groups spent much time in the late 1980s and 1990s going from one legislative battle to the next. It began to appear more sensible to simply regulate tobacco products like other drugs or hazardous products. The tobacco industry benefited from an approach to regulation that essentially said they could do anything that was not specifically forbidden. Given the nature of the product and the legislative precedents for other products, it made more sense to reverse the onus. Tobacco products and the marketing and labeling of these products could be like pharmaceuticals—banned except to the extent that a regulatory authority gives specific permission for specified actions. This was the philosophy behind the new Tobacco Act.

Thinking Globally—Acting Locally

Canada's total consumption of tobacco products represents less than 1 percent of global sales. Although significant progress has been made in Canada, it is only of global significance when it helps efforts in other countries. Similarly, successful measures in other countries can assist efforts to achieve breakthroughs in Canada.

Much of what has happened in Canada has accordingly been done with an eye to global relevance. Many of the key Canadian advocates of tobacco control have long been involved in working at a global level, and much of what has been accomplished in Canada has been immediately communicated in various ways to colleagues elsewhere in the hope of aiding their work.

But the learning goes both ways. Interaction at a global level has greatly assisted Canadian efforts. Not only were Canadians able to learn from the tobacco control initiatives of other countries, but also success in exporting Canadian breakthroughs to other countries reinforced the momentum for continued progress within Canada. For decisionmakers in Canada the moves elsewhere to smoke-free airlines, bigger health warnings on packages, and higher taxes—often with direct connections to what had already happened in Canada—reinforced the sense that Canada was on the right track.

Finding Allies

One of the most intriguing lessons was that although some allies came from expected sources, such as the CCS, other health and medical organizations were simply not comfortable putting much time, personnel, or resources into tobacco control. Indeed, many organizations that represented health professionals who daily saw the devastation caused by tobacco, and many charities dedicated to battling illnesses caused to a large degree by tobacco use, were often only peripheral players in the major tobacco control campaigns.

But other strong allies were constantly being found. Some were dedicated individuals who could rally the support of various constituencies. Individual volunteers with health charities and medical associations were often pivotal in the campaigns. There were also some tremendously engaged ministers of health—politicians who, once they knew they could truly make a difference, literally risked their political futures in efforts to put through public health measures. More than one minister threatened resignation if an equivocating cabinet sided with the tobacco lobby at critical moments in the battles for legislation.

Assistants to politicians, and particularly aides to ministers, were key allies. Usually young, energetic, and idealistic, many of them were committed to ensuring that health measures made it through the labyrinth-like structure of government. They were often the key driving force in getting precedents set, and they seldom received any public acknowledgment of their tremendous efforts.

Doing a Lot on a Limited Budget

Health advocates in Canada seldom had much by way of financial resources. Most campaigns were run on energy and creativity in place of money. Money was always an area in which the tobacco lobby had a huge edge. The health lobby, however, had a relative advantage in its ability to move quickly and creatively.

Many of the major battles cost little or nothing. Volunteers played a huge role in many of the tobacco control victories. Persuading a senior CCS volunteer or prominent physician to speak to a politician was free. Getting information to millions of Canadians through effective media work cost little or nothing. Finding tobacco billboards next to schools simply meant having someone willing to drive around cities and note the location of the signs. Preparing detailed submissions on tobacco taxes often required no more than having someone willing to crunch numbers and present the findings in ways designed to get the attention of a desired audience.

Money helps. But having a lot of money is not a prerequisite for success. Canadian advocates could joke in the 1980s that they were "changing the world on five dollars a day." The formula for success in Canada has involved dedicated action by a variety of actors: strong commitment by municipal, provincial, territorial and federal governments, both politicians and civil servants; good research; and leadership by NGOs that added specialized political and economic research to existing medical and public health research and used it to target public policy and conduct media advocacy campaigns. With the use of new and existing alliances and of grassroots mobilization, these activities were effective with more or less all national political parties. Political ideology played only a minor role in these events, and the tobacco control coalition wisely was usually careful to maintain a nonpartisan stance.

To sum up, it is not a stretch to say that a few individuals in the coalition, working with politicians, the federal bureaucracy, and the media, have potentially saved thousands of lives. This is one of the most important public health stories in Canada's history.

Appendix: Key Dates in Tobacco Control in Canada

1908: Canadian Parliament passes the Tobacco Restraint Act, which prohibits the sale of tobacco products to persons less than 16 years of age.
1951: National Cancer Institute of Canada says there is a possible link between smoking and cancer.

1963: Federal Health Minister Judy LaMarsh states that smoking causes lung cancer.

1963: Tobacco lobby (Canadian Tobacco Manufacturers' Council) is established.

1968: Health Minister John Munroe condemns the advertising of tobacco products.

1974: Non-Smokers' Rights Association is established.

1986: Canadian Cancer Society embarks on public policy advocacy for tobacco control.

1988: Parliament passes Tobacco Products Control Act and the Non-Smokers Health Act.

1991: Federal tobacco taxes are increased by CA$6 (US$5) a carton.

1993: Parliament passes Tobacco Sales to Young Persons Act.

1994: Federal government cuts tobacco taxes in half.

1995: Supreme Court of Canada rules major portions of Tobacco Products Control Act unconstitutional.

1997: Parliament passes the Tobacco Act.

2000: New pictorial health warnings become law.

References

Canadian Cancer Society (CCS), National Cancer Institute of Canada, Statistics Canada, Provincial/Territorial Cancer Registries, and Health Canada. 2001. *Canadian Cancer Statistics, 2001.* Toronto. Available at <http://www.cancer.ca>.

———. 2002. *Canadian Cancer Statistics, 2002.* Toronto. Available at <http://www.cancer.ca>.

Environics Research Group Ltd. 1990. "Awareness of Health Hazards Due to Smoking." December. Prepared for the Canadian Council on Smoking and Health. Ottawa.

Globe and Mail. 1985. "Ontario to Lose $130 Million in Cigarette Taxes." November 2.

Health Canada. 1991. "Canadians and Smoking: An Update." Cat. no. H39-214/1991E. Health Canada, Minister of Supply and Services, Ottawa.

May, N. 1988. "Health versus Big Tobacco: A Review of the Campaign to Pass Bill C-71, the Tobacco Act." Canadian Cancer Society, Toronto.

NSRA (Non-Smokers' Rights Association). 1986. *A Catalogue of Deception.* Toronto.

———. 1992. "The Canadian Tobacco Tax Project." Toronto.

———. 1994. "The Smuggling of Tobacco Products: Lesson from Canada." Toronto.

Rothmans. 1964. "Annual Report." Rothmans of Pall Mall Canada Limited, Toronto.

Statistics Canada. 1991. "Canadians and Smoking: An Update." *Health and Welfare Canada.* Ottawa.

———. n.d. Cat. nos. 32-022-XIB 91-002, 91-512, 91-213. Ottawa.

———. 1994. "Survey on Canada." Ottawa.

Sweanor, D. 1985. "A Review of Tobacco Taxation Policies in the Current Ontario Budget." NSRA, Toronto.

World Bank. 1999. *Curbing the Epidemic: Governments and the Economics of Tobacco Control.* Development in Practice series. Washington, D.C.

5

Democracy and Health: Tobacco Control in Poland

Witold Zatoński

At the end of the 1980s, Poland had the highest cigarette consumption in the world. Polish men, in particular, had been heavy smokers for years. Their addiction had made cancers common and lives short (figure 5.1). By 1990, the odds that a 15-year-old Polish boy would live to the age of 60 were lower than for his peers in most other countries in the world, including India and China (Murray and Lopez 1994). The World Health Organization (WHO) estimated that almost half of the premature deaths among Polish men were caused by inhaling tobacco smoke (Peto and others 1992). Over half of the burden of noncommunicable disease among Polish men was smoking related.

The medical community in Poland began to raise the alarm in the 1980s, when it became clear that the incidence of lung cancer in Poland was higher than almost anywhere else in Europe except Hungary (Zatoński and others 1996). The health, economic, and social costs of smoking spurred Polish doctors and health advocates to look for ways of reversing the advancing health catastrophe.

Tobacco Consumption in Poland: Historical Background

Cigarette smoking accounts for nearly 100 percent of tobacco consumption in Poland. In the 1920s and 1930s tobacco consumption remained stable at a relatively low level of about 500 to 700 cigarettes per person per year. After World War II, the figure rose steadily until the late 1970s, when it was one of the highest in the world, at well over 3,500 cigarettes per person per year (Zatoński and Becker 1988). The economic crisis of the late 1970s limited access to cigarettes, and tobacco consumption stopped rising.

The earliest studies on the prevalence of smoking in different sociodemographic groups date from 1974. The Maria Sklodowska-Curie Memorial Cancer Centre and Institute of Oncology (referred to in this chapter as the Cancer Centre and Institute) in Warsaw has conducted such studies almost every year since 1980. The studies revealed that in the mid-1970s,

Figure 5.1. Probability of Dying of Various Causes for Men Age 15–59, by Region, 1990

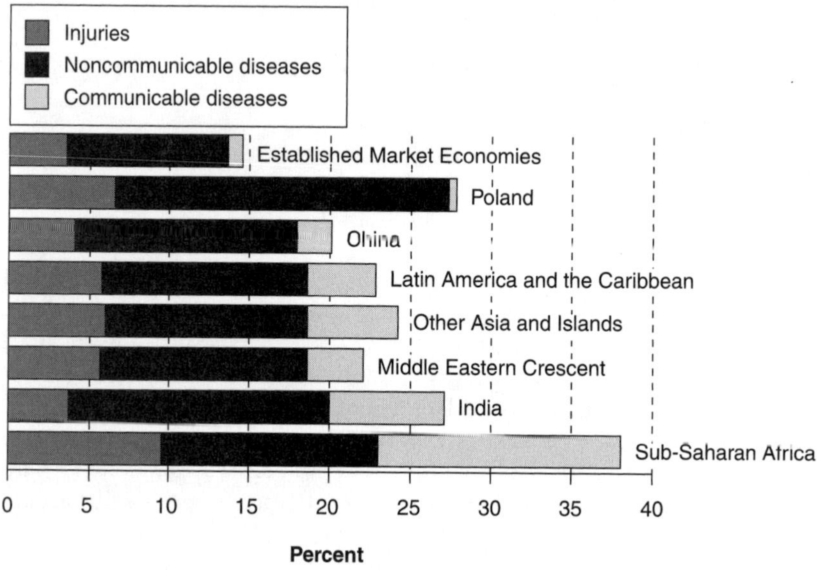

Source: Adapted from Murray and Lopez (1994).

65 to 75 percent of Polish men between ages 20 and 60 smoked every day, and less than 10 percent of men in some age groups said that they had never smoked (Zatoński and Przewoźniak 1992a, 1999). Smokers rarely quit: only a small proportion of men said they were ex-smokers. Smoking was a social norm in the adult male population. Far fewer women smoked than men, but the figures for women also rose consistently for all age groups. From 1974 to 1982, smoking prevalence among adult women increased from 20 to 30 percent—which was the highest level ever recorded (Zatoński and Przewoźniak 1992a). Some of the increase in smoking prevalence was a result of the way that cigarettes were rationed from 1981 to 1983: all employees received a quota of cigarettes whether or not they smoked. The result was an increase of 1 million in the number of smokers between 1981 and 1982, even though the number of cigarettes available on the market was static.

Throughout the 1980s, smoking prevalence among men continued to be very high, although minor decreases were noted in all age groups and more people in the youngest group began reporting that they had never smoked. This change may have been due to limited availability of cigarettes. The percentage of women smoking remained at about 30 percent, but considerable differences appeared across age groups. Smoking prevalence among the oldest women was 5 to 10 percent, compared with nearly 50 percent among the youngest adult women (Zatoński and Przewoźniak 1999).

Tobacco-Related Diseases

The growth of tobacco consumption in Poland after World War II led to an increase in morbidity and mortality caused by diseases and disorders related to inhalation of cigarette smoke. Lung cancer is a good indicator of health damage caused by smoking because it is found almost exclusively among tobacco smokers (Tyczyński and others 2000). After World War II, lung cancer mortality in Poland increased for men and women in all age groups. In the mid-1960s it was relatively low compared with rates in the United Kingdom and the United States (figure 5.2). In middle-aged men, however, lung cancer mortality increased rapidly. By the late 1970s it exceeded rates in both the United Kingdom and the United States (figure 5.3), and it continued to climb in Poland well after it had dropped in the other two countries (Zatoński 1995). The health consequences of inhaling cigarette smoke were less marked for women because of lower smoking prevalence (Peto and others 1994).

By the early 1980s the incidence of lung cancer among middle-aged Polish men was among the highest in the world and was significantly higher than it had ever been in any high-risk Western European country (for example, the United Kingdom or Finland). Figures for other cancers related to the inhalation of cigarette smoke, such as laryngeal and oral cancer, had also reached their highest levels by that time. Six of the 10 most frequent cancer sites in men were tobacco related (Zatoński and Tyczyński 1997). Epidemiological estimates indicate that 58 percent of malignant tumors in middle-aged men were caused by cigarette smoking. Similarly, studies showed that 42 percent of cardiovascular deaths and 71 percent of respiratory disease mortality among middle-aged men were smoking related (Peto and others 1994).

Tobacco Control in the 1980s

Unlike the case in most developed and developing countries, information about tobacco-related health damage was censored in Poland. Tobacco and cigarette production was an important source of government revenue. Health and the factors determining health were given little prominence in the media, which were controlled by the totalitarian regime. Scientific reports on health damage from tobacco smoke that received publicity in Western countries did not reach Poles. Public awareness of the dangers of tobacco use remained low.

Figure 5.2. Mortality Trends for Lung Cancer, All Age Groups, Men and Women, Poland, the United Kingdom, and the United States, 1959–99

Men

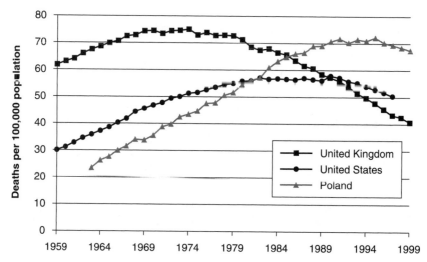

Women

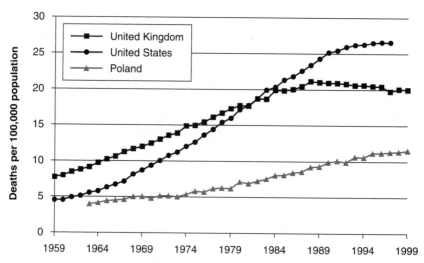

Source: Cancer Centre and Institute, Warsaw, using data from Peto and others (1994) and Central Statistical Office of Poland (various years).

Figure 5.3. Mortality Trends for Lung Cancer, Men Age 45–64, Poland, the United Kingdom, and the United States, 1959–99

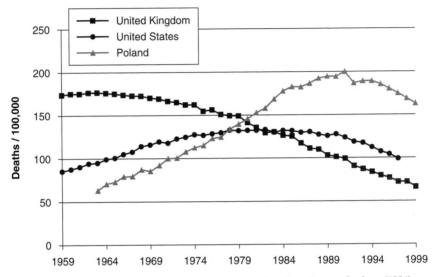

Source: Cancer Centre and Institute, Warsaw, using data from Peto and others (1994) and Central Statistical Office of Poland (various years).

Existing tobacco control regulations were paper tigers—they looked strong on paper but were ineffective because of lack of enforcement. For example, a 1974 law forbidding smoking in health centers was never enforced. This was a problem of considerable importance because cigarette smoking by physicians in health centers became widespread. In some medical specialties the percentage of doctors who smoked was higher than among the general population. In fact, physician smokers outnumbered all Polish women smokers.

New Information about Tobacco

The growing catastrophe in adult health was first described in the early 1980s, as the voice of Polish civil society, symbolized by the democratic Solidarity movement, was gaining influence. As Polish society gradually became more open, more information on health issues was aired in the media. The 1980s saw the first publication of general information and scientific papers documenting tobacco smoking as the key causal factor in the growing cancer epidemic and in premature mortality among young and middle-aged adults (see, for example, Zatoński, Gottesman, and Przewoźniak 1987).

The political changes of the 1980s made possible the establishment of public organizations intent on improving the health of Poles by reducing the popularity of smoking. Several groups associated with the medical profession launched scientific studies, as well as activities that included developing tobacco control programs, educating the public, organizing debates and scientific conferences, and establishing links with international organizations. Through those international contacts, especially with the International Union against Cancer (UICC) and the WHO, Polish health advocates became involved in actions to reduce tobacco consumption.

In the early 1980s the Cancer Centre and Institute undertook systematic studies on the health consequences of cigarette smoking in Poland. Within a framework of international cooperation, investigators used WHO standard methodologies and definitions to document the relationship between smoking and the rapidly growing cancer epidemic. From these studies came the scientific basis for the first Polish report on smoking and health in Poland (Zatoński and Przewoźniak 1992a, 1992b).

Also in the early 1980s, the medical and scientific communities organized the first scientific conferences and workshops, in collaboration with the UICC and with Finnish medical organizations. These gatherings contributed to the growing understanding of the magnitude of smoking-related disease in Poland. They also highlighted the potential for effective interventions. During this period, health experts from Finland (Matti Rimpelä) and the United Kingdom (Richard Peto and Michael Wood) helped develop the first research and intervention programs.

While this scientific and public health activity was going on, tobacco control advocates began communicating their message to the public with the help of the media. They also organized Poland's first participation in World No Tobacco Day, in collaboration with the WHO.

Advances Despite Constraints

These efforts did not always receive government support and were sometimes criticized by government officials. In the early 1980s the prime minister's legislative council rejected a bill, prepared with the help of experts from Finland and the UICC, that would have established regulations to help reduce the health consequences of smoking. Officially, the bill was dropped on technicalities, but the actual reason was the perceived threat it posed to the country's weak economy. The tobacco sector was a government monopoly, and it was feared that a reduction in smoking would affect government revenues.

Similarly, attempts to alert the public, whether at home or abroad, to Poland's poor health conditions could be only partly successful. Free media did not exist in Poland, and the government had little interest in health matters. In a nondemocratic system, health-related activities could be implemented only to a limited extent unless they were supported by the government.

Despite limited government support, tobacco control advocates made the 1980s an important period of preparing scientific assessments, compiling databases, training experts, establishing links with international organizations, and developing intervention programs. They took advantage of their opportunities and achieved four important things:

- The creation of a body of independent experts
- The establishment of the Polish Anti-Tobacco Society, an organization of health advocates
- The initiation of scientific research to document, for the first time, the role of tobacco in the adult health crisis in Poland
- The initiation of collaboration with scientific, social, and international organizations abroad.

The Impact of Democracy and a Free Market

With the breakdown of the communist system, Polish tobacco control advocates faced new challenges and opportunities. Regulations governing economic activity were changed to make way for a free market in 1988 and 1989. The introduction of a market economy seemed likely to increase tobacco use, with grim consequences for public health. The production and sale of cigarettes, which had been entirely controlled by the government, was one of the first economic sectors to be privatized. Within a few years, the Polish tobacco companies were taken over by multinational corporations, and by the end of the 1990s, more than 90 percent of the country's tobacco industry belonged to multinationals.

An almost immediate result of privatization was the unrestrained availability and improved consumer appeal of cigarettes. All international brands could now be found on the domestic market, together with new local brands such as Solidarność (Solidarity), Lady Di, Sobieski (named for a famous Polish king), and George Sand. Privatization also led to a rapid shift away from reliance on tobacco grown in Poland, and this, together with the introduction of modern equipment, caused a considerable reduction in the workforce. With the construction of new and technically more advanced factories, the industry's productivity increased substantially.

In the rapid privatization, the authorities made considerable concessions to the multinational companies, such as agreeing to keep tobacco taxes low for several years. As a result, the real prices of cigarettes remained low throughout the first half of the 1990s: a pack of one of the cheapest brands cost less than a loaf of bread. Higher

tobacco taxes that raised cigarette prices were levied only in the second half of the 1990s. Even so, at the end of the 1990s the tax rate was
only 47 percent, while in European Union (EU) countries the minimum
rate was 57 percent.

The Tobacco Lobby Moves into Action

The multinational tobacco companies developed a lobby to promote their
interests. An important part of their efforts involved establishing good
relations with the emerging class of politicians, particularly economic and
financial specialists. For example, the tobacco lobby made a donation to
Lech Wałęsa, then leader of the Solidarity trade union, in hopes of gaining his support.

As soon as they entered the Polish market, transnational tobacco companies worked to undermine the traditional ban on tobacco advertising.
They were unable to overturn the internal regulations against tobacco
advertising on national television (there were no private television channels at the time), but they did manage to overcome restrictions in all other
media, including public radio and the press, the first of the media to be
privatized. The tobacco companies introduced advertising techniques
that Poles had never before experienced. The industry soon became the
largest advertiser in the country; toward the end of the 1990s it was
spending US$100 million a year on advertising cigarettes in Poland
(National Association of the Tobacco Industry 1998).

The unfamiliar marketing techniques had a powerful effect on a receptive public. The decrease in the prevalence of smoking halted, and the
number and percentage of occasional smokers rose. The most important
change was a surge in the number of children experimenting with cigarettes, with a particularly dramatic increase in the number of girls who
smoked. The percentage of girls between the ages of 11 and 15 who
smoked at least once a week increased from 16 percent in 1990 to 28 percent in 1998 (Mazur, Woynarowska, and Kowalewska 2000).

The opening of the market, the takeover of Polish tobacco companies
by the multinationals, and the use of state-of-the-art marketing techniques all appeared to have determined the future of the tobacco epidemic in Poland. The industry set itself a goal of increasing tobacco consumption by about 10 percent over 10 years. Predictions concerning
health were pessimistic. The evidence of increasing premature mortality
among young and middle-aged adults between 1988 and 1991 seemed to
confirm such fears (Zatoński 1995).

These growing health threats were challenges for health advocates. But
democracy, an emerging civil society, and independent, news-craving
mass media also opened up new opportunities for action.

The Kazimierz Declaration

Even before the political system changed in most Eastern European countries, Poland hosted a conference at Kazimierz in November 1990 with the title "A Tobacco-Free New Europe." The Cancer Centre and Institute organized the conference under the honorary patronage of Lech Wałęsa, the historic Solidarity leader, and in collaboration with the UICC and the American Cancer Society. It was the first meeting of health advocates from Western and Eastern Europe aimed at taking action to close the health gap between the two parts of the continent. It was also the first opportunity to present comprehensive scientific evidence on the magnitude of the health damage caused by smoking in Eastern Europe.

The conference targeted public health leaders from Eastern European countries. Many of the participants later became national leaders in tobacco-and-health policy in their own countries. Other participants included representatives of leading international health organizations such as the WHO and experts on tobacco and health from Europe and the United States, including Richard Peto of Oxford University; Greg Connolly of the Massachusetts Department of Health, director of one of the biggest tobacco control programs in the world; and Michael Wood from Belfast, then director of the UICC's Program on Tobacco and Cancer.

The conference ended with the endorsement of the Kazimierz Declaration, which recommended that national governments adopt comprehensive tobacco control programs to reduce the health consequences of cigarette smoking. The declaration emphasized that in a democratic state, legislation was the key to curbing the damage to health from smoking. It recommended that governments take the following steps:

- Introduce and enforce a strict ban on all direct or indirect advertising and promotion of tobacco goods or trademarks
- Adopt, as a minimum, EU standards for health warnings on cigarette packs
- Adopt, as a minimum, EU standards for maximum tar deliveries but with delays to allow national tobacco manufacturers to comply with maximum levels of 20 milligrams by 1995 and 15 milligrams by 2000
- Ban the introduction of smokeless tobacco and any new forms of tobacco
- Impose a substantial health surcharge on all tobacco products to raise the minimum price of cigarettes
- Regularly monitor tobacco-related mortality and smoking prevalence
- Immediately establish national tobacco control coordinating committees
- Recognize the need for smoke-free public environments

- Educate the public, especially young people, about the hazards of tobacco use
- Support smokers who want to stop smoking.

The Kazimierz conference also provided a framework for cooperation in tobacco control among Central and Eastern European countries. Not long after the conference, the WHO Collaborating Centre on the Action Plan for a Tobacco-Free Europe was set up at the Department of Epidemiology and Cancer Prevention of the Cancer Centre and Institute. Through it, Poland became a center for educating and training public health leaders in Central and Eastern Europe.

The Kazimierz Declaration provided a basis for health-related tobacco control action in Poland in the 1990s. Polish public health advocates saw the Kazimierz conference as a milestone in formulating objectives and as a catalyst for work on a parliamentary bill to reduce cigarette smoking with the goal of improving the health of the Polish people. Not surprisingly, the international tobacco industry viewed the conference with anxiety.

Establishment of the Health Promotion Foundation

In the new political milieu, nongovernmental institutions could be set up to achieve public goals. The Health Promotion Foundation was established to organize and support health promotion activities aimed at preventing smoking-related diseases and increasing consumption of fruits and vegetables.[1] Its continuing activities include:

- Developing and offering education programs
- Supporting scientific research
- Cooperating with local and international organizations such as the UICC and the WHO
- Organizing and making presentations at conferences and workshops.

The foundation's tour de force has been a mass campaign to help smokers quit. This drive takes place every autumn, climaxing on the third Thursday in November. Its Polish name can be translated as the Great Polish Smoke-Out, and it is based on the Great American Smoke-Out campaign. Within a few years, it became the largest regular public health campaign in Poland. Originally centrally organized, the campaign now relies on the active involvement of local communities and local media.

---

1. The foundation was set up by the author. Its limited budget comes from private donors, and its project funding, from international and other organizations. Its work is greatly facilitated by a strong partnership with Polish media.

Studies tracing the campaign's impact year by year have shown that 80 to 90 percent of Poles have heard of it. Many smokers credit the campaign with inspiring them to smoke less or stop smoking (Jaworski, Przewoźniak, and Zatoński 2000):

- Every year, 20 to 30 percent of smokers have tried to smoke less.
- Every year, about 1 million smokers (out of about 9 million daily smokers) have attempted to quit smoking.
- Every year, 200,000 to 400,000 people claim to have quit smoking thanks to the campaign.

Over more than a decade of campaigns, more than 2 million people have successfully quit smoking for good. These impressive results testify to the campaign's importance in improving the health of Poles.

Part of the campaign's success comes from a popular annual competition. All Poles who have quit smoking since the beginning of the year can take part simply by sending in postcards to the Health Promotion Foundation. The competition has become more popular each year, and in 2000, the 10th year, more than 40,000 postcards were submitted. The prize, awarded to a number of randomly chosen participants, is a one-week stay in Rome, including a private audience with Polish-born Pope John Paul II.

Both public and commercial media support the program, with public radio and television being the main media sponsors. Every year, thousands of news items describe the campaign. Special advertisements, information on how to quit, discussions, and reports are broadcast and printed. The competition and the trip to Rome traditionally receive wide television coverage.

New Legislation for Tobacco Control

In 1989 the upper chamber of Parliament, the Senate, became the first democratically elected political institution in postwar Poland. Because of their high social status, medical professionals formed an unusually high proportion of senators. Consequently, health advocates chose to begin legislative action in the Senate.

Soon after the Kazimierz conference, a working group at the Cancer Centre and Institute developed a preliminary draft of a tobacco control bill, together with a statement of reasons for approving it. The health-related arguments presented were backed up with scientific evidence, which included the dramatic level of premature mortality in Poland caused by inhaling cigarette smoke. The bill was based on WHO standards for good tobacco control legislation and included a comprehensive set of provisions for reducing cigarette consumption.

Politicians, and especially the medical professionals holding senatorial posts, welcomed the draft bill. A working group headed by Dr. Maciej Krzakowski of Cieszyn was formed in 1991 to prepare the motion. Soon afterward, the bill was introduced in the Senate.

Controversy Over the Proposed Bill

To the surprise of politicians and health advocates, the bill encountered strong opposition from the tobacco lobby. For the first time in the new democratic era, politicians were faced with the activities of a well-organized interest group determined to achieve its goals.

The controversy over the bill soon became public. The health of Poles and the harm done by cigarette smoke became the subject of a stormy public debate lasting many years. The media, now independent, but not always free of external influences, played a key role in the debate. The health evidence was irrefutable—which is not to say that the tobacco industry has never questioned it. The discussion therefore centered on whether legislation (which is, after all, a piece of paper) could improve the health of a nation.

Cigarette companies tried to make parliamentarians (and the entire nation) believe that the legislation would be ineffective. They questioned the efficacy of an advertising ban, health warnings, economic regulations, and education, and they referred to freedom of advertising. Above all, they warned that a ban would have a negative impact on Poland's future economic development.

Initially, the media and public opinion were skeptical about the need for the legislation. What seemed to turn public opinion was the consistent argument by health advocates that smoking was largely responsible for the catastrophic state of the health of adult Poles. In the last stage of the debate, opponents of the bill, now losing ground, concentrated their attack on the proposed advertising ban. The maintenance of the right to advertise cigarette products became a key area of possible compromise.

On the government side, financial decisionmakers disagreed with the proposal to allocate some tobacco tax revenue for financing actions to improve health by reducing smoking. In general, however, support for the legislation was rising among politicians and the public, irrespective of political affiliation. Public attitudes toward smoking were changing. The ongoing public debate had drawn the attention of Poles to the health costs of smoking, and they were also becoming more aware of reduced tolerance for smoking in other countries. As public awareness increased, political parties took notice.

The Bill Passes

In a country where democracy was only beginning to take root, a succession of short-lived governments might have been vulnerable to the efforts of the tobacco lobby to derail the bill. The industry encouraged the use of a presidential veto and, failing at that, sought at least to delay the passage of the bill as long as possible. But no matter which political party dominated Parliament, the work and the debate on tobacco control legislation continued. On November 9, 1995, the Law for the Protection of Public Health against the Effects of Tobacco Use passed with an overwhelming majority (90 percent) of votes from all political parties.

Some of the key areas covered by the new act were

- Smoking bans in health care establishments, in schools and other educational facilities, and in closed spaces in workplaces.
- A ban on selling tobacco products to minors under 18.
- A ban on selling tobacco products in health care establishments, schools and other educational facilities, and sports facilities.
- A ban on selling tobacco products in vending machines.
- A ban on producing or marketing smokeless tobacco products.
- A total ban on advertising tobacco products in electronic media (radio and television).
- Restrictions on advertising in other media. (Advertisements in print media and on billboards had to carry health warnings in the upper part of each advertisement, occupying 20 percent of the area.)
- Publication of health warnings on all cigarette packs. (The warnings were to occupy 30 percent of two of the largest sides of each pack.)
- Free provision of treatment for smoking dependence.

With the exception of two areas—lack of a total advertising ban and of a fund dedicated to improving smokers' health—the new law included all the actions outlined in the WHO's gold standard for tobacco control. The Polish legislation effectively provided for the protection of non-smokers and introduced the world's largest health warnings on cigarette packs. It also obligated the government to prepare annual action programs for controlling the health consequences of cigarette smoking. Implementation reports have been presented to Parliament every year since then.

The new regulations were enforced without much trouble, although there were some technical problems. For example, no company or industrial enterprise had a separate ventilated room to allocate for smokers' use. As a result, the regulation on implementing this measure only became effective after five years; the provision of special rooms finally became a requirement on January 1, 2001. Within a short time, many workplaces, particularly in the private sector, became truly smoke-free, allowing smoking only in specially designated places.

The Industry Strikes Back

Having succeeded in preventing a total ban on tobacco advertising, the tobacco lobby immediately launched an aggressive campaign against the placement of large health warnings on cigarette packs. The lobby maintained that the new legislation was inconsistent with current EU regulations and would hinder Poland's admission to the EU. Industry officials feared that these health warnings, the first to be introduced in a European country, would create a precedent.

They were right. A few years later, the European Parliament referred to the Polish example as it began action to implement even larger health warnings on cigarette packs sold in EU countries. Warnings that occupy 30 to 40 percent of the two larger sides of a cigarette pack are being introduced in the EU in 2003.

A pro-tobacco parliamentary lobby was mobilized on an unprecedented scale to try and thwart the plans to introduce the health warnings. Many Polish politicians regard the scope and intensity of that lobby as the most powerful in the entire first decade of parliamentary democracy in the country. For health advocates, the offensive against the existing legislation provided another opportunity to call the public's attention to the health catastrophe resulting from cigarette smoke.

The fight of the tobacco industry's Goliath against the health advocates' David came under intense scrutiny in the media and even received international coverage. Undaunted by successive defeats, the tobacco lobby made three attempts to change the 1995 legislation during the *vacatio legis* (the period between the promulgation and the implementation of a law). The last attempt, a few months before the 1997 elections, was marked by a vigorous debate that almost resulted in a physical fight in Parliament. In spite of the enormous political and financial effort, on April 11, 1997, the tobacco lobby lost the battle to change the size of health warnings on cigarette packs. This time, however, the majority was small: 148 in favor, 122 against, and 100 abstentions.

In mid-1998, after two and a half years of negotiations, Parliament finally confirmed that health warnings on cigarette packs sold in Poland were to occupy 30 percent of the two larger sides of the pack. These were the largest warnings in the world until Canada introduced larger, pictorial warnings in 2001.

Figure 5.4. Nominal and Real Trends in Tobacco Excise Taxes and Average Monthly Salaries, Poland, 1993–2002

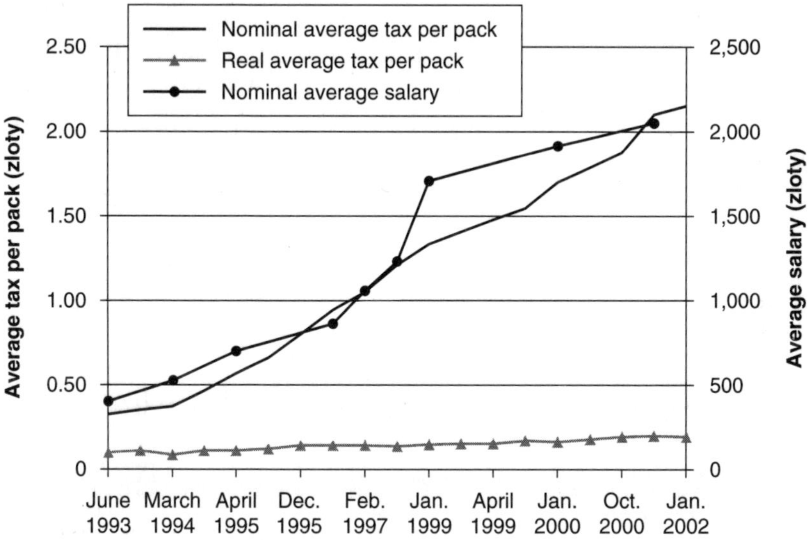

Source: Cancer Centre and Institute, Warsaw.

The Role of Cigarette Pricing

In privatization agreements concluded in the early 1990s, the government had agreed to freeze tobacco taxes. As a result, in the first half of the 1990s increases in cigarette prices remained below the inflation rate (which was high at the time), and taxes on cigarettes never exceeded 30 percent of the retail price, compared with the EU minimum of 57 percent and an EU average of about 75 percent. Increases in nominal cigarette prices matched income growth, and so cigarettes become increasingly affordable throughout the decade (figure 5.4).

The 1995 act stipulated that the government must take effective economic action through a pricing policy designed to limit tobacco use. In 1997 health advocates began collaborating with the World Bank and the University of Chicago to investigate the economics of smoking in Poland. The work included analyzing the effect of cigarette taxes and price increases on smoking behavior (see, for example, Zatoński, Matusiak, and Przewoźniak 1998). The preliminary results of this analysis showed that higher taxes and higher cigarette prices would result in a decrease in the number of cigarettes smoked and an increase in total tax revenues. Only when these results were presented did the rate of tobacco tax increases accelerate. In 1999 and 2000 the tax on tobacco products increased by approximately 30 percent each year. It must be stressed that this economic tool—higher taxes that raise prices—has a particularly strong impact on less well-educated and poorer people. This is often the group with the highest smoking prevalence and the least likelihood of quitting in response to information about the harmful health effects of smoking (World Bank 1999). Unfortunately, not all politicians and economists are convinced of the effectiveness or advisability of using prices as a tool for limiting tobacco use.

Advertising Back on the Agenda

In 1998 a newly elected Parliament moved tobacco advertising onto the agenda once again. Parliamentarians were alarmed by new evidence showing a decrease in the age at which children (especially girls) begin smoking (Mazur, Woynarowska, and Kowalewska 2000). They were also responding to growing public concern about aggressive advertising by tobacco companies, which Poles regarded as being targeted mostly at children. There was a general consensus that these two factors—the growing popularity of smoking among children and aggressive cigarette advertising—were directly related and could be changed by a total ban on cigarette advertising. A new bill was introduced and this time moved rapidly through Parliament. A total ban on tobacco advertising was passed on September 10, 1999, by a large majority: 374 in favor, 11 against, and 12 abstentions. All political parties endorsed the bill. The new law included a provision for allocating 0.5 percent of tobacco excise tax revenue to the National Tobacco Program with the aim of reducing the health consequences of smoking. By December 2000, tobacco advertisements had been removed from billboards all over the country. Since 2001, tobacco advertising has been banned in all print media.

The progress of this bill, the parliamentary debate, and the media commentaries reflected the change in Polish society's attitude toward smoking. The decrease in smoking prevalence and the interest among smokers in trying to quit are striking. International studies indicate that the climate in Poland for health improvement through reducing tobacco consumption is one of the most favorable in Europe (Fagerström and others 2001).

Democracy Is Healthier

Democracy and a free-market economy have turned health into an important value in personal and family welfare in Poland. Pro-health behavior, the growing share in the Polish diet of vegetables and fruits (now available in great variety all year round), the popularity of a Mediterranean diet, and sports—all are at odds with inhaling tobacco smoke. The change in attitude toward smoking is most noticeable among educated Poles who have more experience of life in other countries, especially in the United States, and are aware of a lack of tolerance there toward smoking. In certain communities, being a nonsmoker has become fashionable, and smoking no longer receives social approval. Quitting smoking is a popular New Year's resolution.

Local and religious communities have become an important setting for discussions about the health effects of smoking. The Catholic Church is the main sponsor of the annual November antismoking campaign, and it also encourages nonsmoking at the local level—for example, when priests meet with engaged couples. Schools are also active in health promotion, helping to increase awareness of the dangers of tobacco use. The activities are aimed at parents, as well as at students and teachers.

Consumption Drops Dramatically

In the 1990s sales figures for cigarettes in Poland decreased for the first time since World War II. Tobacco industry data show that cigarette consumption fell by 10 percent between 1990 and 1998 (Michaels 1999). This reduction was achieved when the market was functioning normally and despite the enormously aggressive advertising policies of the tobacco companies. (As noted above, in the late 1990s the tobacco industry was spending US$100 million annually on advertising.)

The drop in cigarette consumption was the result of reduced smoking prevalence in many different groups in society (Zatoński and others 2000). As figure 5.5 shows, smoking prevalence among men decreased in all age groups between 1975 and 1999. For women, a reduction in the popularity of cigarette smoking has been observed mainly in the younger age groups. The least significant reductions and the highest smoking prevalence are among middle-aged Poles of both genders, with no decline in prevalence evident (yet?) among middle-aged women. The overall decrease in smoking is most marked among better educated groups; among less well-educated Poles, the decrease in smoking is much less.

To sum up, smoking in Poland peaked at the end of the 1970s, with approximately 14 million smokers. At that time, 62 percent of all adult men and 30 percent of adult women smoked, and percentages for many age groups were higher. Prevalence levels remained at these levels in the 1980s but decreased substantially in the 1990s. At present, slightly fewer than 10 million Poles smoke—about 40 percent of adult Polish men and a little more than 20 percent of adult Polish women.

Figure 5.5. Smoking Prevalence by Age Group, Men and Women, Poland, 1975, 1985, and 1999

Men

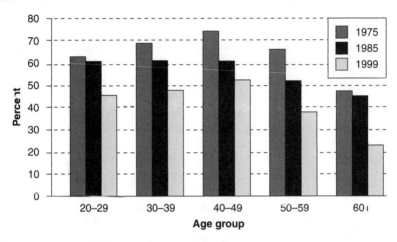

Women

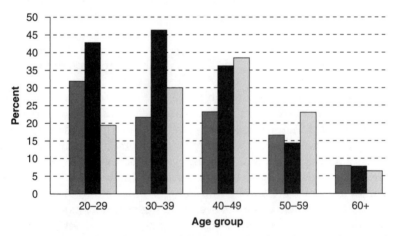

Source: Cancer Centre and Institute, Warsaw, using data from the Central Statistical Office of Poland (various years).

Health Indicators Improve

The drop in smoking across much of the Polish population has improved the country's health indicators. As noted at the beginning of this chapter, the incidence of lung cancer is the best and most specific measure of changes in exposure to tobacco smoke. In Poland shifts in this epidemiological indicator clearly reflect the history of exposure of the Polish population to cigarette smoke.

The upward trend in lung cancer mortality in the youngest age group of adult men (age 20–44) was reversed in the 1980s, and by the end of the 1990s mortality had decreased by about 30 percent from the peak level. A 19 percent decline in lung cancer mortality in middle-aged men (age 45–64) followed in the early 1990s. In the over-65 population, the effects of the changes in exposure to cigarette smoke are still not evident.

In Hungary trends in lung cancer incidence before 1980 were similar to those in Poland. Hungary has not implemented effective tobacco control measures, and unlike the trend in Poland, the incidence of lung cancer is still increasing. The current incidence figures in Hungary are the highest ever for young and middle-aged adult men and women. In the United States and the United Kingdom, by contrast, trends in the epidemiology of lung cancer resemble those observed in Poland, although over a different time period (see figure 5.2, above).

Paralleling the changes in lung cancer mortality in Poland are decreasing mortality trends for other tobacco-related cancers, such as those of the oral cavity, larynx, and pancreas (Zatoński and Tyczyński 1997). Another positive change since 1991 has been a significant 20 percent reduction in cardiovascular disease (Zatoński, McMichael, and Powles 1998). About 10 to 40 percent of all cardiovascular disease in Poland is estimated to be tobacco-related. (The range reflects age-group and gender differences.) Exposure to cigarette smoke plays a less important role in cardiovascular disease than in lung cancer, but some of the decrease in cardiovascular disease is probably due to reduced exposure to cigarette smoke.

The reduction in smoking in Poland in the 1990s was also a factor in the drop in infant death risk during that decade. The lower risk is related to a decrease in the percentage of infants with low birth weight (<2,500 g)—from 8.4 percent in 1989 to 5.9 percent in 1999 (Szamotulska and others 2000). An estimated 20 to 30 percent of the reduction in risk can be attributed to lower exposure to cigarette smoke among pregnant women and their unborn and newborn babies. Between 1985 and 1999, the prevalence of smoking among women age 20–29 dropped significantly, by about 23 percent.

Overall, the total mortality rate in the Polish population from all causes fell by about 10 percent between 1991 and 2000, corresponding to a decrease of nearly 36,000 deaths annually. The reduction in cigarette consumption is estimated to be responsible for about one-third of the reduction in mortality across all age groups, or about 10,000 deaths a year (Zatoński 2000). Life expectancy—the best overall health indicator—increased in the 1990s by almost four years for men and almost three years for women.

Lessons Learned

Despite the significant progress in the past decade, Poland's journey toward health improvement through tobacco control is just beginning. The experience gained in these early stages will provide the foundation for future strategies.

Strong Warnings Have an Impact

One focus of early efforts has been on increasing public awareness of the health hazards of smoking. A valuable tool in raising awareness has been the large, clear warnings on cigarette packs. As a result of the introduction of the warnings, 3 percent of smokers stopped smoking, 16 percent attempted to quit, and another 16 percent are now more aware of the harm done by smoking (Zatoński, Przewoźniak, and Porębski 2000).

Pricing Policy Is Key, Especially for the Health of People with Low Incomes

The message about the harmful effects of cigarette smoke has mainly influenced better-educated Poles. Among people with basic education, including pregnant women, smoking prevalence has decreased very little (Zatoński and Przewoźniak 1999). Cigarette prices have been rising at a slower pace than incomes, which makes cigarettes more affordable and tends to increase consumption, especially among lower-income groups.

Pricing policy is an area of strategic importance for further limiting the health consequences of cigarette smoking. The World Bank's review of evidence shows clearly that it is the strongest and most effective single measure (World Bank 1999), and recent observations in Poland have confirmed this (Czart and others 2000). But the reduction in tobacco consumption that Poland has achieved so far is not attributable to the introduction of a pricing policy, since significant price increases occurred only after 1997. Taxation policy has only just begun to be used to reduce tobacco use in Poland, and more could be done.

Doctors and Other Medical Professionals Need to Do More

Medical advice is another effective method of motivating smokers to quit. Even though the antismoking climate in Poland is one of the most favorable in Europe, the contribution of physicians and other medical professionals to treating tobacco-dependence syndrome remains insignificant. Only 2 to 3 percent of ex-smokers report medical assistance in quitting.

Polish ex-smokers are mostly those who were the least addicted. Nearly one-half of daily smokers (about 4 million) smoke their first cigarette within the first half-hour after waking up. In the most addicted cases, 8 percent of adult male smokers and 4 percent of adult female smokers (a total of 0.5 million people) wake up during the night to smoke a cigarette (Zatoński and Przewoźniak 1999).

The smokers with the strongest addiction and the greatest exposure to cigarette smoke are those born between 1940 and 1960. They reached adolescence (and started smoking) between 1955 and 1975, a period of widespread social acceptance of smoking. Smokers in this group either already suffer from severe smoking-related health problems or will before long see symptoms of the health damage caused by their smoking. This group should receive special medical attention and should be the target of carefully designed immediate interventions. Stopping exposure to cigarette smoke always brings substantial health benefits, even after many years of smoking (Peto 2002).

Nicotine addiction is a medical problem, so supporting those who want to quit or have quit is a special task for physicians. Both general practitioners and specialists (cardiologists, pulmonologists, obstetricians, pediatricians, and oncologists) should be made aware that helping people cure their tobacco addiction is part of a doctor's responsibility to his or her patients. It is impossible to cure patients of major diseases, such as chronic bronchitis and cardiovascular diseases, including coronary heart disease, without first getting them to quit smoking. Health providers in Poland are becoming more involved in helping patients stop. Some health insurance policies cover treatment to help people stop smoking, which makes economic sense, since smokers have much higher annual health care costs than nonsmokers.

Another great challenge in Poland that demands immediate action and a long-term campaign is reduction of pre- and postnatal exposure to tobacco smoke. Smoking during pregnancy and exposure of young children to cigarette smoke remain problems. In fetal and infant life, secondhand smoke is an important contributing factor to poor health. Intervention programs supported by local communities should be undertaken to protect children from this risk.

Science-Based Evidence Is Important to Justify Action

In all of Poland's tobacco control efforts, solid scientific evidence has played a key role. It has helped convince the general public of the dangers of tobacco consumption and has provided the justification for programs and legislation.

The Polish experience in changing people's attitudes toward smoking shows the dominant role of medical evidence. This evidence, based chiefly on domestic data compiled in collaboration with leading research centers abroad under the auspices of the WHO, demonstrated the extent of the epidemic of diseases caused by inhaling cigarette smoke. In particular, highlighting the causal relationship between cigarette smoke and cancers, especially lung cancer, proved to be a good tactic. People viewed news on this link as reliable because the information came from the national Cancer Centre and Institute and was endorsed by prominent scientists. The ready acceptance of this information in the late 1980s may have been the result of increased awareness of the problem as the epidemic of tobacco-related diseases reached its peak. Poles were able to compare the health messages and scientific evidence with news about the health of their relatives and friends who were smokers.

Legislation Is Essential for Progress in Tobacco Control

Another important contribution to Poland's progress in tobacco control has been the legislation enacted in 1995 and 1999. The years 1990 to 1995, in particular, when the tobacco control law was drafted, were crucial to the later success of tobacco control efforts. Especially effective was the debate surrounding the bill, when the public heard the strong health evidence against smoking and observed the tobacco industry's actions to prevent the bill from being passed. The process of introducing and defending the legislation provided a forum for changing public attitudes toward tobacco, especially among the best-educated groups of society.

One important lesson from the Polish experience in preparing the bill is that legislative tactics must correspond to the level of public awareness of the issue. In the early 1990s Poles did not understand the importance of a total ban on tobacco advertising for reducing the health consequences of tobacco smoking. Only after years of watching the practices of the tobacco industry and following the national debate did people change their attitudes. This is reflected in the initial rejection of the total advertising ban in 1995 and its adoption in 1999 by an overwhelming majority of votes and with support from all political parties.

Both the 1995 legislation and its 1999 amendment have proved instrumental in changing the attitude of Poles toward tobacco use. Still, this transformation should be viewed as a phased process rather than a revolutionary change. Large, clear health warnings on cigarette packs that stigmatize the product, a ban on smoking in public places, and a total ban on tobacco advertising help reinforce this attitudinal change day after day.

Local Involvement in Tobacco Control Efforts Is Crucial

Rapid further progress in tobacco control is not possible without the involvement of local communities. In recent years activity regarding tobacco control has been transferred from the Parliament and the central government to local communities. The attitudes and participation of local role models have become ever more important in supporting tobacco control activities. Involvement of local health providers is crucial in the battle against tobacco-related diseases.

Despite all these achievements, several thousand Polish smokers still die needlessly and prematurely every year because of smoking. Tobacco control continues to be a health priority in Poland.

References

Central Statistical Office of Poland. Various years, 1945–99. *Statistical Yearbooks* (in Polish). Warsaw.

Czart, K., S. Matusiak, F. Chaloupka, K. Przewoźniak, and W. Zatoński. 2000. "What Influences Smoking in Poland? Impact of Tobacco Taxes and Smoker Income" (in Polish). In "Abstracts of the Second National Scientific Conference on Smoking and Health, Warsaw, November 15, 2000." *Alkoholizm i Narkomania* 13 (3): 424–25.

Fagerström, K. O., P. Boyle, M. Kunze, and W. Zatonski. 2001. "The Anti-Smoking Climate in EU Countries and Poland." *Lung Cancer* 32 (1): 1–5.

Jaworski, J. M., K. Przewoźniak, and W. Zatoński. 2000. "The Great Polish Smoke-Out 1991–1999 and Its Impact on Smoking Behaviours in Adult Population." In "Second Conference on Health Status of Central and Eastern European Populations after Transition, June 5–7, 2000, Warsaw, Poland." *Abstracts:* 204. Maria Sklodowska-Curie Memorial Cancer Centre and Institute of Oncology, Warsaw.

Mazur, J., B. Woynarowska, and A. Kowalewska. 2000. "Tobacco Smoking: Health of School-Aged Children in Poland" (in Polish). Faculty of Psychology, University of Warsaw.

Michaels, D. 1999. "Targeting Poles Who Smoke like Chimneys: Activists Make Headway in Fight against Tobacco Use." *The Wall Street Journal* (April 8).

Murray, C., and A. Lopez. 1994. "Global and Regional Cause-of-Death Patterns in 1990." *Bulletin of the World Health Organization* 72 (3): 447–80.

National Association of the Tobacco Industry. 1998. "Tobacco Advertising. Facts." Warsaw.

Peto, R. 2002. Keynote speech at WHO European Ministerial Conference for a Tobacco-Free Europe, February, Warsaw.

Peto, R., A. Lopez, J. Boreham, M. Thun, and C. Heath Jr. 1992. "Mortality from Tobacco in Developed Countries: Indirect Estimates from National Vital Statistics." *Lancet* 339: 1268–78.

———. 1994. *Mortality from Tobacco in Developed Countries 1950–2000.* Oxford, U.K.: Oxford University Press.

Szamotulska, K., K. Przewoźniak, M. Porębski, and W. Zatoński. 2000. "Infant Mortality in Poland in the Nineties. II. Decrease of the Prevalence of Low Birth Weight—Change in Behavior: Smoking." In "Second Conference on Health Status of Central and Eastern European Populations after Transition, June 5–7, 2000, Warsaw, Poland." *Abstracts:* 183. Maria Sklodowska-Curie Memorial Cancer Centre and Institute of Oncology, Warsaw.

Tyczyński, J., U. Wojciechowska, J. Didkowska, and W. Zatoński. 2000. "Deaths Due to Smoking in Poland in the 1990s." In "Eleventh World Conference on

Tobacco or Health—Promoting a Future Without Tobacco, August 6–11, 2000, Chicago, Ill." *Abstracts*, vol. 2: 377.

World Bank. 1999. *Curbing the Epidemic: Governments and the Economics of Tobacco Control.* Development in Practice series. Washington, D.C.

Zatoński, W. 1995. "The Health of the Polish Population." *Public Health Review* 23: 139–56.

———. 2000. "Development of the Health Situation in Poland in Comparison with Other Countries of Central and Eastern Europe" (in Polish). Maria Sklodowska-Curie Memorial Cancer Centre and Institute of Oncology, Warsaw.

Zatoński, W., and N. Becker. 1988. *Atlas of Cancer Mortality in Poland 1975–1979.* Berlin. Springer Verlag.

Zatoński, W., and K. Przewoźniak. 1992a. "Tobacco Smoking in Poland." In W. Zatoński and K. Przewoźniak, eds., *Health Consequences of Tobacco Smoking in Poland* (in Polish), 29–44. Warsaw: Ariel.

———. 1992b. "Selected Harmful Substances in Polish Cigarettes." In W. Zatoński and K. Przewoźniak, eds., *Health Consequences of Tobacco Smoking in Poland* (in Polish), 75–86. Warsaw: Ariel.

———. 1999. "Tobacco Smoking in Poland: Attitudes, Health Consequences and Prevention" (in Polish). Maria Sklodowska-Curie Memorial Cancer Centre and Institute of Oncology, Warsaw.

Zatoński, W., and J. Tyczyński, eds. 1997. *Epidemiology of Cancer in Poland 1980–1994* (in Polish). Warsaw: Maria Sklodowska-Curie Memorial Cancer Centre and Institute of Oncology.

Zatoński, W., K. Gottesman, and K. Przewoźniak. 1987. "Smoking and Malignant Neoplasm Mortality in Poland" (in Polish). *Pneumonologia Polska* 55 (7–8): 357–61.

Zatoński, W., S. Matusiak, and K. Przewoźniak. 1998. "The Need for Tobacco Control in Poland." In I. Abedjan, R. Van Der Merve, N. Wilkins, and P. Jha, eds., *The Economics of Tobacco Control: Towards an Optimal Policy Mix*, Section 3: *Country Case Studies in Tobacco Control*, 282–92. University of Cape Town, South Africa.

Zatoński, W., A. J. McMichael, and J. W. Powles. 1998. "Ecological Study of Reasons for Sharp Decline in Mortality from Ischaemic Heart Disease in Poland since 1991." *British Medical Journal* 316 (7137): 1047–51.

Zatoński, W., K. Przewoźniak, and M. Porębski. 2000. "Large Cigarette Pack Warnings Change Smoking Behaviours in Poland." In "Workshop and Poster Session on Challenges to Tobacco Control for Eastern Europe in the 21st Century, August 8, 2000. Eleventh World Conference on Tobacco or Health—Promoting a Future Without Tobacco, August 6–11, 2000, Chicago, Ill." *Abstracts:* vol. 3: 777.

Zatoński, W., M. Smans, J. Tyczyński, P. Boyle, in collaboration with N. Becker, J. Didkowska, H. P. Friedl, J. Holub, Z. Peter, I. Plesko, V. Roman, R. Stabenow, and C. Tzvetansky. 1996. *Atlas of Cancer Mortality in Central Europe.* IARC Scientific Publications 134. Lyon, France: International Agency for Research on Cancer.

Zatoński, W., K. Przewoźniak, M. Porębski, U. Wojciechowska, W. Tarkowski, and E. Harville. 2000. "The Smoking Decline in Poland: Does It Apply to All Socioeconomic Classes?" In "Workshop and Poster Session on Challenges to Tobacco Control for Eastern Europe in the 21st Century, August 8, 2000. Eleventh World Conference on Tobacco or Health—Promoting a Future Without Tobacco, August 6–11, 2000, Chicago, Ill." *Abstracts:* 50.

6
Political Change in South Africa: New Tobacco Control and Public Health Policies

Mia Malan and Rosemary Leaver

Over the past decade, there has been a dramatic turnaround in the South African government's attitude toward tobacco control. Before 1993, tobacco control policy was virtually nonexistent, but the 1999 Tobacco Control Amendment Act gave the country some of the most progressive tobacco control policies in the world.

Today, all tobacco advertisements and sponsorships have been banned; smoking at work and in restaurants is illegal, except in clearly demarcated areas; and explicit health warnings are required on all cigarette packs. Although cigarettes are still relatively cheap in South Africa, excise taxes represent almost 50 percent of their total retail price, after significant increases in 1994 and again after 1997 (van Walbeek 2002b).

As a result of these policies, cigarette consumption is on a downward spiral. According to Corné van Walbeek of the School of Economics, University of Cape Town, it decreased from 1.9 billion packs in 1991 to about 1.3 billion packs in 2002. The rate of decline has accelerated especially since 1997, when large tax increases sharply increased the price of cigarettes. In light of these accomplishments, many today regard South Africa as a model for other countries.

But these gains have not come easily. They are the result of decades of steadfast lobbying by the health community and antismoking groups and of the new South African government's commitment to public health. And they have come in the face of vehement opposition from the tobacco industry, advertising agencies, hospitality associations, and, until the early 1990s, an apartheid government with extraordinarily close links to the trade itself.

The History: Early Days, Early Struggles

As long ago as September 1963, the *South African Medical Journal,* in a far-sighted editorial, offered advice to the health minister of the time:

There should be no hesitation about banning smoking in public places and on public transport. . . . Cigarette advertising should at first be restricted as to quantity and content with a view to its eventual limitation. It might also be advisable to insist that each cigarette packet should carry a notice to the effect that the contents are potentially dangerous to health. The minister of health may also attempt further restrictions of smoking by increasing the taxation on cigarettes. . . . The matter is important and urgent.

Dr. Yussuf Saloojee, executive director of the National Council Against Smoking (NCAS), has ironically remarked that these suggestions were considered so "important and urgent" that 12 years passed before a single one of them was acted on (Saloojee 1993a). In 1975 the tobacco industry volunteered not to advertise cigarettes on television, but it took another 12 years for it to agree to print on cigarette packs a warning ("Smoking is a health risk.") that was "vaguely worded, badly placed and in very small print" (*Hansard* 1993).

"A Crime of Apartheid"

Some have maintained that the government's historical lack of interest in tobacco control was "a crime of apartheid," arguing that the tobacco industry was dominated by white, Afrikaans-speaking South Africans with very close ties to the government (Wilkins 2000). The history of the tobacco industry in the country, particularly prior to 1993, bears out this view.

The tobacco manufacturing industry in South Africa is very highly concentrated. The Rembrandt group used to control 87 percent of the market, with British American Tobacco South Africa (BAT) being the only other company with any significant market share. Under the able leadership of the Afrikaner businessman Anton Rupert, Rembrandt developed into a very successful corporation, and it is often perceived as a symbol of the Afrikaans-speaking community's rise to economic power. After its merger with Rothmans International, it gained control of 95 percent of the market. Rupert retained a strong hand through his control of two companies, Remgro and Richemont, that owned 30 percent of BAT.

Rupert became one of the most powerful businessmen in South Africa: he built up strong links with virtually every major decisionmaker, including legal firms and media institutions, and was on the board of most major trusts. Yach (2002) recalls that "anywhere you turned in the media and tried to get a story published that advocated tobacco control, you were blocked by their absolute fear and trepidation of Rupert's long reach through his tobacco companies." Ironically, Rupert's wife was involved with South Africa's Cancer Association, while her husband's products were killing many of the people she was fighting to keep alive (Yach 2002).

Rembrandt had a long history of backing the National Party, which was dominated by Afrikaans-speaking South Africans. The two were, in fact, founded in the same year, 1948, and "grew up together" (Yach 2002). The National Party represented Afrikaner political power, and an unhealthily close relationship between the tobacco industry and the government had far-reaching implications for policymaking.

In the early 1990s Rembrandt rebuilt one of then-president F. W. de Klerk's homes, and there were annual Rembrandt-funded outings for cabinet ministers. For its part, the National Party government demonstrated a favorable attitude toward the industry through low excise taxes, virtually unrestrained advertising, and an absence of restrictions on smoking in public places. For instance, within party circles, it was well-known that F. W. de Klerk's predecessor, P. W. Botha, strongly disliked smoking—so much so that he forbade it at cabinet meetings. Yet Botha never expressed his attitude in antitobacco measures (Perlman 1991a).

During this time, the tobacco industry (in effect, Rembrandt) was the Ministry of Finance's prime adviser on cigarette excise matters, with no indication of any Ministry of Health influence. This was clearly reflected in Finance Minister Barend du Plessis' 1983 budget speech, when he warned, "The Tobacco Board has presented justified arguments for the maintenance of the status quo regarding the excise taxes on tobacco and I do not intend to wake sleeping dogs." Three years later, in 1986, du Plessis again refused to increase excise taxes on cigarettes, arguing that any tax increase could adversely affect consumption and lead to a reduction of revenue (van Walbeek 2002a).

At the time, excise taxes accounted for less than 30 percent of the retail price, and the real excise rate on tobacco had been decreasing steadily for the previous 15 years, eroded by inflation. It is hard to imagine that the minister's grasp of basic economics was so flawed that he believed his own statement. He, like his peers in many countries around the world, would have known very well that a tax rate increase would in fact lead to an *increase* in revenues. The decrease in consumption in response to a price increase would be smaller in percentage terms than the tax rise. The higher tax revenues per pack would generate higher total revenues, despite a somewhat lower sales volume.

The Cape Town Debate

The effect on policy of the relationship between the government and the tobacco industry became evident in 1989, when the Cape Town City Council announced plans to restrict cigarette advertising and smoking in public places. In protest, Rembrandt threatened to withdraw its sponsorship of the Cape Town Symphony Orchestra. The company's influence went well beyond its sponsorship: it commanded an enormous network of power and influence, and there was a significant threat of retribution if its wishes were thwarted. Rembrandt's tactic worked: Kobus Meiring, the administrator of the Cape Province, refused to pass the legislation needed to enforce the council's plans (Dennehy 1989a).

The restrictions, which had been proposed by Dr. Michael Popkiss, Cape Town's chief medical officer, would have required restaurants to set aside at least half their tables for nonsmokers (Doman 1989a). Existing by-laws outlawed smoking only on the lower decks of buses, in cinemas, and in public elevators. New restrictions on tobacco advertising were also proposed: in addition to the ban on cigarette commercials on television, cigarette advertising would be prohibited in all council-owned buildings and properties (Dennehy 1989a).

Four days before the council debate on the proposal, Popkiss wrote to Anton Rupert appealing for funds for an AIDS awareness campaign. An outraged Rupert turned down the request, saying that his refusal came "from an industry you have decided to destroy" (Bateman 1989b) in pursuit of "not only dictatorial, but clearly impracticable" objectives (Morris 1989). The exchange prompted Cape Town mayor Peter Muller to rebuke Popkiss for his insensitivity and bad timing, declaring that he found it "incongruous that the [medical officer] can write a financial appeal only four days before a major smoking debate—he must either think that Dr. Rupert is foolish, or alternatively, he's totally devoid of any sensitivity" (Bateman 1989b). Muller's chastisement was immensely embarrassing to the medical officer, as it was highly irregular for a mayor to publicly rebuke a city official.

At the council debate, strong support was shown for the proposal, with 25 councillors voting in favor and only 5, including the Cape Town mayor himself, against. A palpable discomfort existed, however, between Popkiss and the administrator and mayor. This tension was exacerbated by the leak of internal correspondence between Rupert and Popkiss in which the Rembrandt chair accused Popkiss of being "hell-bent to create new regulations against the freedom of the individual to decide for himself" (Bateman 1989b). To worsen the situation, there was a further leak of a letter from the mayor to the council's executive committee in which he was highly critical of Popkiss and his suggested regulations.

The publicity surrounding this feud sparked a heated debate in the letters pages of Cape Town newspapers. The National Council Against Smoking, the Heart Foundation, the Cancer Association, and the Medical Association of South Africa sprang to Popkiss's defense, praising him for creating awareness about the health hazards of smoking and pledging their full support for the bylaw.

The restaurant industry, which had remained silent until then, began actively voicing its concerns. A local organization, the Cape Restaurateurs

Association, gave the council 12 days to withdraw the bylaw or face the threat of court action. When the Cape Town council refused to oblige, the association issued a summons, stating that the ban was "irregular, ultra vires, invalid and unreasonable" (Doman 1989a). The Federation of Hotel, Liquor and Catering Associations of South Africa (FEDHASA) organized a petition signed by 307 Cape Town restaurants to protest the new bylaw. The restaurateurs' primary objections were that the bylaw infringed on their right to decide how best to run their businesses (Doman 1989a) and that some restaurants were too small to be reasonably expected to divide their eating areas (Leaver 2002). The Cape Town Chamber of Commerce did not remain silent either: it argued that business in South Africa was already overregulated and that "efforts should be directed toward doing away with regulations rather than devising more ways to inhibit business activity" (Cape Town Chamber of Commerce 1990).

Against the fierce opposition to the bill, the health lobby made a compelling case based on the health hazards posed by smoking and inhaling secondhand smoke. And a large majority of the Cape Town public supported restrictions on smoking in enclosed public spaces. The bylaw was only one step away from becoming effective when it was vetoed by Cape Province administrator Meiring. In response, Popkiss commented that he "had never been in favor of the 50–50 rule anyway, because [it] had not been shown to protect non-smokers" (Leaver 2002).

The Evidence against Tobacco Mounts

Meanwhile, a small success was achieved in a different arena. Key players in the public health community, including Prof. Harry Seftel, then at the Medical School of the University of Witwatersrand, and Drs. Derek Yach and Krisela Steyn of the Medical Research Council, were compiling evidence on the harm caused by tobacco in South Africa and on the high costs that tobacco use imposed on both the state and patients in the form of treatment costs for tobacco-related illnesses, forgone earnings, and premature deaths.

As early as 1982, Yach published one of the first tobacco control articles in the *South African Medical Journal*. His study was considered so controversial that the Medical Research Council refused to publish it under its own name but instead listed it as a personal contribution. The study focused on the economic aspects of smoking in South Africa, claiming that "while it is true that a reduction in tobacco and cigarette production would cause some losses to the national economy and individuals, it is also true that the reduction in total costs accompanying such a decrease would more than compensate these losses" (Yach 1982). Encouraging authors to publish studies under their own names was "a

highly exceptional stance to take," indicative of even the medical establishment's fear of "the impact of negative reactions of tobacco companies" (Yach 2002).

But the persistent efforts of Yach and his colleagues eventually paid off.
In 1988 they succeeded in arranging a special "tobacco focus" issue of the
South African Medical Journal, to coincide with the first World No Tobacco
Day. It was the first time ever that an entire issue of the *Journal* had been
devoted to one preventive aspect of public health, and it was considered
a major breakthrough in tobacco control. Yach described it as a critical
turning point because "we were not just saying the deaths were rising, we
started getting a projection of what was going to happen in the future and
introduced the fact that there were practical legislative options that had
been taken around the world." The *Journal* had a huge impact in South
Africa, receiving extensive coverage and discussion and helping set a
basis for future action. So, the publication of the special issue was a first
step toward "bridging the gap between epidemiological data sitting in
scientific journals and popularizing the data in the mass media and
among political groups" (Yach 2002).

The high medical costs of treating smoking-related illnesses at hospitals were drawn to the public's attention. In an editorial in the *South
African Medical Journal,* Anton Rupert was accused of using "emotive language" to obscure facts, including the fact that "smoking caused almost
half of the cases at Groote Schuur, Cape Town's premier hospital" (Bateman 1989b). These realities did not elude authorities at the University of
Cape Town, who used the hospital as a training facility. In March 1989
smoking and the sale of cigarettes were banned in all public areas of the
medical school campus, including cafeterias and bars (*Cape Argus* 1989b).

As political opportunities emerged in later years, the strong evidence
base helped support and justify actions. Yach (2002) saw the first indication of success in 1991, when initial documents of the new African
National Congress (ANC) government's Reconstruction and Development Plan strongly featured tobacco control as an intended policy. It was
helpful that a number of people who eventually assumed senior positions in the government had become colleagues of Yach and Steyn in the
Medical Research Council in the years just prior to the turnover of power.
The most prominent of these were Dr. Nkosazana Zuma, who was health
minister from 1994 to 1999, and Dr. Olive Shisana, who became director-
general of health in 1995.

Action and Reaction: Efforts Elsewhere

Where Cape Town had failed, Johannesburg dared to tread. In March 1991
the Johannesburg City Council banned smoking in take-away restaurants

and required that 60 percent of seating in all other eateries be reserved for nonsmokers (Burgers 1991). The council faced strong opposition from pro-tobacco groups such as the Johannesburg Chamber of Commerce (Woodgate 1991), but it stood by its decision, arguing that council members would rather have "egg on their faces than death on their consciences" (Nevill and Gill 1991).

Steps had also been taken in the Eastern Cape Province, where the medical officer of Port Elizabeth had banned smoking in prominent public buildings in the city. Even private companies started to act: many declared their cafeterias and boardrooms smoke-free areas and encouraged smoking executives to attend subsidized quit-smoking courses (Barrett 1989).

These events, particularly those in Johannesburg, prompted Popkiss to launch a new offensive against smoking in 1992, asserting that Cape Town should match the bylaw passed in Johannesburg. The Cape Town medical officer was convinced that his new recommendations would fare better than previous ones had, since they were shorter, simpler, and easier to understand. For the second time, however, his proposals came under heavy attack from pro-tobacco lobby groups, and once again the Cape Province administrator refused to pass the bylaw.

A Turning Point

With the second failure to pass a no-smoking bylaw, prospects for legislation in the Cape Province seemed dim. On the national level, however, the appointment of the country's first woman health minister provided a gleam of hope. Dr. Rina Venter may not have been a pro-control advocate when she assumed office, but she was an open-minded social worker with sympathy for nonsmokers who had to suffer from passive smoking (Saloojee 1993a). Perhaps her most important quality was that she was a skilled politician and person of integrity who was prepared to fight for legislation she believed in.

Yussuf Saloojee remarked that "the spark that may have served to focus the mind of the minister on the issue" came in 1991, in the debate on her first health budget (Saloojee 1993a). During the discussion, an opposition member of Parliament, Carole Charlewood, criticized the government, accusing it of "protecting the vested interests of the powerful tobacco industry, and not the people of the country." Charlewood's attack was based on the 1988 report of the Medical Research Council, "Smoking and Health in South Africa: The Need for Action" (Yach and Townsend 1988), which argued that "the costs of the tobacco industry to society outweighed its benefits" (Wilkins 2000) and advocated strong measures to discourage smoking.

Venter knew that, other than low-key, low-budget educational campaigns, the government had very little with which to defend itself against
Charlewood's accusations. In her reply the health minister therefore
promised to look into the possibility of tobacco control legislation. She
later said that "she regarded the matter as sufficiently important to make
the decision there and then without having first consulted with her cabinet colleagues" (Saloojee 2002). According to Saloojee, that moment was
the turning point in the administration's approach to tobacco control: "It
was a vital public commitment, and the first signal of new thinking on
this issue at the highest levels of government."

Building Support

Venter was well aware of her party's vested interests, and she recognized
that it would be unrealistic to expect full support for her plans. She also
knew that one minister, however determined, was "not going to disperse
the smoke ring alone" (Perlman 1991a). The outcome of her undertaking
would depend crucially on how much support the health department got
from the rest of the government. It was not only her party's well-oiled links
with the industry that seemed to stand in her way: the state president and
many of his colleagues were chain-smokers. In fact, when F. W. de Klerk
was asked to observe No Tobacco Day by not smoking, his office replied
that his schedule that day was too stressful for him to do without (Perlman
1991a). But despite being a heavy smoker, de Klerk knew that the addiction
was harmful, and he supported moderate measures to discourage smoking.

The tobacco industry was a major source of taxes, export revenue, and
jobs. According to Perlman (1991a), in 1990 the industry generated 988 million South African rand in taxes, employed over 60,000 people, and spent
nearly 90 million rand on advertising.[1] There were, furthermore, several
major tobacco-sponsored sports events such as Benson & Hedges cricket
and the Rothmans July Handicap, the premier horse race.

But Venter had a strategy. Shortly after her announcement, one of the
country's most influential antitobacco alliances, the Tobacco Action
Group (TAG), sought a meeting with her. TAG consisted of three large,
highly vocal lobbying organizations: the Heart Foundation of Southern
Africa, the Cancer Association of South Africa, and the National Council
Against Smoking. TAG was highly effective in using "public fora and the
media to warn the public against the dangers of tobacco, to call on the
government to introduce effective counter measures, and to discredit the
industry's claims about their product and the importance of their indus-

1. In 1991, 2.5 South African rand = 1 U.S. dollar.

try" (van Walbeek 2002a). Venter knew that she would not be able to steer a tobacco control bill through Parliament without positive media coverage and outside support. She therefore made a pact with the alliance: she would push for a draft bill from inside if TAG would see to matters outside the legislature (Saloojee 1993a). Saloojee later remarked that Venter "stood by her word throughout this process" (Saloojee 2002).

The agreement meant that the health minister did not have to spend time campaigning for favorable media coverage and backing beyond Parliament: experts were going to do it for her. This plan fit well with the changing role tobacco-control lobbyists saw for themselves during the early 1990s: "Rather than lobbying the policymakers, they were working with the policymakers in publicizing the positive aspects of the proposed tobacco measures" (van Walbeek 2002a).

But however skilled TAG was, it did not face an easy task. The country's two most powerful media institutions at the time, the South African Broadcasting Corporation (SABC) and Nasionale Pers, had close ties with the tobacco industry and were in many respects government controlled. Nasionale Pers owned almost all Afrikaans newspapers and had sold a considerable proportion of its company shares to Rembrandt (Perlman 1991a). The SABC received substantial government subsidies and claimed that many of its radio stations could not survive without cigarette advertisements (Saloojee 1993a).

When the NCAS produced its first antismoking commercial, which it regarded as "a first step towards educating the public to stop being seduced by cigarette advertising" (Levy 1991a), the SABC refused to broadcast it. The corporation conceded that it had a gentlemen's agreement with the cigarette companies, saying that "because the tobacco industry had voluntarily undertaken not to advertise tobacco products on TV, it would be unfair to accept anti-smoking ads" (Levy 1991b). In stark contrast with other print media companies, Nasionale Pers was (unsurprisingly) reluctant to place the advertisement and coyly said it wanted to look at the copy before deciding. The visual broadcast version of the commercial, entitled "Smoky Conversation," showed six young people picnicking and smoking in an idyllic setting while talking about the dangers of their addiction. It was to be shown in all major cinemas for two weeks in April that year, but at a high and unusual cost: Cinemark, one of the country's biggest cinema chains, waived its usual policy of presenting public service messages gratis and charged for showing it. The reason was clear—fear of losing tobacco advertising, as almost a third of all cinema ads were for cigarettes (Perlman 1991a).

Saloojee dismissed the SABC's stance as "rubbish." Tobacco was "undeniably the largest preventable cause of death and the NCAS had a right and a duty to inform the public about its dangers using all available media."

The industry declined to comment, arguing that "smoking was too emotionally loaded to be put into perspective in a single paragraph" (*East London Daily Dispatch* 1991). Instead, it released a leaflet, "Common Sense in Smoking—Personal Choice and Moderation the Key" (Perlman 1991a), which asserted that allegations against smoking were based on heated reactions rather than factual foundations. One paragraph stated, "The industry does not react to points of view which are made merely for the sake of generating publicity, but prefers to put its own point of view to those people who are mindful of their health and the convenience of others and who are prepared to make allowances for other forms of enjoyment."

When the industry called for private talks with the minister, it became apparent that it had more than the distribution of pamphlets planned: it was going to spend sizable amounts to fly in three international consultants to persuade the minister that legislation was unnecessary (Saloojee 1993a). Venter agreed to the meeting provided that she could involve local tobacco control advocates, including TAG, the Medical Research Council, and an economist from the University of Cape Town. Two years later, during the proceedings of the Extended Public Committee, she described the encounter: "We spent an entire afternoon, from two o'clock to five o'clock, on this matter. These people gave an elucidation of research which in their opinion, as they interpreted it, indicated that tobacco smoke was not at all harmful" (*Hansard* 1993).

Saloojee (2002) recalls an apprehensiveness within the tobacco control group, some of whose members "felt like the 'B' team, and were slightly intimidated by the international experts." But in the end, the South Africans were the ones who convinced the minister. At the conclusion of the meeting, Venter "unequivocally stated that she was going to proceed with legislation because it was her department's duty to warn smokers of the risks of smoking and to protect the rights of non-smokers without infringing on the rights of smokers" (Saloojee 1993a).

Yet again, there was a strategy involved. Yach recalled that

> the minister instructed us to be on our worst possible behavior, which was quite pleasant to be. I'm pretty sure they thought they were coming into a developing country where the knowledge base about the tobacco industry's behavior was poor. But we had already been fully briefed—through our links with international colleagues—on everybody who was going to be before us. We knew all their arguments and that they could be countered easily. (Yach 2002)

Venter later described it as a day of great satisfaction:

> If there has been one day in my life on which I have been proud of our scientists, it was that day. Not only did they testify to the thoroughness

with which they do research, but also demonstrated that they could hold their own in a debate on an international level in which arguments were being advanced in regard to the harmfulness or otherwise to one's health of tobacco smoke. (*Hansard* 1993)

Saloojee believed "the industry's ability to buy expensive foreign lobbying consultants" had turned into a liability: "Nationalism became an advocacy tool. It was a matter of national pride that the home-grown scientists had put the foreign experts in their places" (Saloojee 1993a).

The Road to Legislation

Months later in 1991, Venter introduced the Control of Smoking and Advertising of Tobacco Products Draft Bill. The proposed legislation would give her powers to bar or limit smoking in certain public places and make it an offense to sell cigarettes to anyone under 16. But the real sting was in the changes the minister wanted to make to the advertising code for tobacco products: visual commercials would be required to carry a rotating health warning, and broadcast versions would have to include the phrase "smoking is a health risk" in a voice similar to that of the main presenter of the advertisement (Perlman 1991a). Advertisements would not be allowed to:

- Depict any woman of childbearing age as being associated with smoking
- Imply that smoking is associated with success in sports
- Imply that the use of tobacco products is a sign or proof of manliness, courage, or daring or enhances feminine charm.

Restrictions were also to be placed on tobacco companies' sponsorship of sporting events and any other activities implicitly associated with health, success, or youth. Together, these restrictions called almost every cigarette advertisement in South Africa into question.

Tobacco control lobby groups welcomed the proposal but pointed out that a multifaceted approach was needed. The National Council Against Smoking suggested a "comprehensive anti-smoking program centered around increased taxes on tobacco products" (Leaver 2002). The Medical Research Council reiterated this plea, expressing concern about the increased incidence of smoking among teenagers in poorer, predominantly black communities (*Medicine Today* 1991). The tobacco industry chose not to comment.

Stumbling Blocks

Venter's draft legislation was to be published in the *Gazette* on June 28, 1991. (All proposed legislation must be published in the *Gazette* before

being introduced in Parliament.) It was at this point that the "vested interests" that Member of Parliament Carole Charlewood had commented on
in 1991 became apparent: a day after Venter had her "triumphant" meeting with the tobacco industry representatives and local antismoking
advocates, the government delayed her plans to publish the proposals.
The state maintained that the delay would allow for "the incorporation of
a few new ideas" and would give the minister time to review them (Perlman 1991b). Authorities promised that the postponement would be minimal. But two months later, in September 1991, the health department
announced that the draft legislation would only be submitted in the following year's parliamentary session.

In March 1992 the proposed law reemerged, this time as the Tobacco
Products Control Bill. TAG immediately organized a workshop to
broaden support for the bill, inviting professional, labor, and community
associations. Each organization was asked to issue a public statement on
smoking and health and to make representations in favor of the legislation. Through this lobbying process, 86 percent of the submissions
received by the Department of National Health and Population Development were in support of the proposals (Saloojee 1993a).

The bill's most significant opponents were the South African Business
Institute and the SABC. TAG felt that there was not much it could do to
influence the Business Institute but that "the opposition of the SABC
could prove a major impediment" (Saloojee 1993a). The SABC asked for
radio to be exempt from broadcasting health warnings, as some of its
radio stations received up to a third of their revenue from cigarette commercials. It argued that the industry would shift its advertising from radio
to billboards and print media, where it could more easily disguise warnings. The SABC's case was strongly argued, and research had shown that
many illiterate people identified cigarettes by package design and would
not understand printed health messages. A compromise was reached that
exempted radio stations provided that they set aside a pro rata amount of
free time for broadcasting health messages.

The tobacco industry yet again refused to comment publicly. It stuck to
its "private approach," with the Tobacco Institute of South Africa (TISA)
sending representatives directly to the health minister (Leaver 2002).

In June 1992 the health department once again announced that the bill
was unlikely to come before Parliament until the next year. Although
Parliament was due to adjourn later that month, the bill was not on the
order paper, nor had it been referred to the Joint Committee on Health
for consideration. A health department spokesperson said the minister
was still discussing the bill with interested parties but strongly denied
rumors that the delay was the result of pressure from tobacco organizations. It later emerged that TISA had been given the opportunity to sub-

mit further representations to the health minister and had met with her earlier that month.

Many of Venter's fellow National Party ministers were in disagreement with the bill. For example, the minister of agriculture criticized what he viewed as "punitive measures " against smokers and saw it as "fitting that the industry had simultaneously tried to improve its position and combat the anti-tobacco lobby by forming the Tobacco Institute of South Africa earlier that year" (Leaver 2002). He emphasized how much revenue the industry provided to the state. Antismoking advocates criticized the minister's failure to mention the costs of tobacco use in the form of disease, lost productivity, and medical expenses to the state, which, a widely publicized Medical Research Council report argued, "far outweighed the benefits of smoking, defined as the sum of tax revenue accruing to government and income earned by employees in the tobacco industry" (Leaver 2002).

Health advocates were also greatly concerned about the delays in the legislation, knowing that the industry would do everything in its power to use the postponements to stop it from being passed. Saloojee remarked that "it was difficult to understand the delay in the bill's publication when the express purpose of publication was to elicit comment" (*Cape Times* 1991).

Political Support from the New Government

One important factor that worked against the tobacco industry was South Africa's changing political landscape. By 1992, the country was in transition; its first democratic elections were only two years away, and Nelson Mandela, the country's president-in-waiting and one of the leaders of the antiapartheid liberation movement, the ANC, had gained considerable support after being released from prison in 1990.

Two months after the draft bill was finally published for comment, on World No Tobacco Day, May 31, 1992, Mandela made his stance on smoking clear when he declared his total support for the bill, appealing to all South Africans to back antitobacco campaigns. Thereafter, the tobacco industry's strategy changed noticeably. Saloojee (1993a) observed that it moved from "trying to defeat the bill, to simply weakening it" and speculated that, after hearing Mandela's statement, the industry realized that killing the bill could result in even stronger legislation from a future ANC government. These conjectures seemed to be confirmed when, shortly after Mandela's statement, cigarette companies complained to the minister that the issue had been politicized, "and that while they could trust the present government, they were not too sure about the next."

Another watershed event was the international conference on tobacco use and its control in Africa that Yach and other members of the Medical Research

Figure 6.1. De Klerk Prepares to Take Leave of Power and the Tobacco Control Debate: A Cartoonist's Perspective.

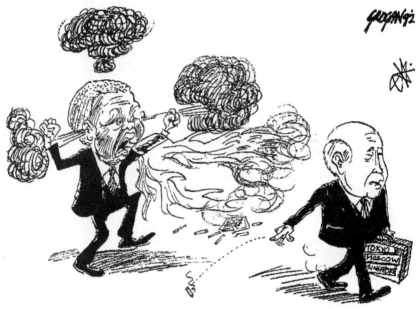

"It would be better for all if you stopped smoking."

State President de Klerk was known to be a heavy smoker but supported weak tobacco control efforts. Future president Mandela had made a strong statement of support for the tobacco control bill, which de Klerk's government was delaying.

Source: Cape Times, June 2, 1992.

Council had long been planning and that finally took place in Harare, Zimbabwe, in 1993. Dr. Nkosazana Zuma, who had recently been hired by the Medical Research Council and was soon to become the first health minister of the new South African government, gave the opening speech in her capacity as a representative of the ANC. She made clear her personal commitment, and her party's commitment, to strong efforts to reduce tobacco use in South Africa. The more than 100 conference participants included a large South African delegation, people from about 35 other countries, several notable international experts in tobacco control, and a small huddle of representatives of tobacco growers (Chapman and others 1994).

Debates in Parliament

In Parliament, which still consisted mostly of National Party members, the tobacco industry maintained its strong influence. The Tobacco Products Control Act was tabled in March 1993, after a delay of more than a year. During the interim, TAG was assured that the bill had been approved with minor changes. Although concerned that it had not been told what these revisions were, the lobbying group saw no reason to make a public issue of this. When TAG finally did get to see the tabled version, it was stunned: "The bill as introduced had been completely watered down. The clause restricting smoking in public places had disappeared, and spoken communications were exempted from the need to broadcast health warnings" (Saloojee 1993a).

It was obvious that the bill had met with considerable resistance in the cabinet, as shown by a telling comment that Hernus Kriel, the minister of law and order, made before the cabinet meeting at which the bill was discussed. He was heard to say loudly that Venter's proposals would never reach Parliament, as "50 percent of the cabinet plus one" would oppose it. When questioned who the "50 percent plus one" were, he replied that the state president was the 50 and he was the "one" (Saloojee 1993a).

The first reaction of tobacco control advocates was to reject the weakened bill, but following extensive deliberations they instead decided to make representations to Parliament to try to strengthen the proposed legislation. TAG, the Medical Research Council, and the Johannesburg and Cape Town City Councils each asked to be allowed to give evidence to the Joint Committee on Health. Cigarette companies sent the Tobacco Institute to do the same, yet again with international experts in tow.

Tobacco control supporters argued that a recent Medical Research Council study had shown that the majority of the public supported tobacco control legislation, that the bill distorted the meaning of the word "advertising" because it did not include radio advertising, and that Parliament would be subject to ridicule if it allowed the legislation to pass (Saloojee 1993a). According to the lobbyists, radio was a major issue, as it reached more South Africans than the other media. Moreover, radio, in contrast to print media, was accessible to the large part of the population that was illiterate—a market in which the industry was showing a growing interest.

Cigarette companies responded by releasing studies disputing the statements of the antismoking lobby. One study, by Health Buildings International, argued that "more workers complained about temperature, stuffiness, and lighting than about tobacco smoke and noise" (Perlman 1993). Other studies cast doubt on the links between smoking and disease or contended that restrictions on tobacco advertising were ineffective (Saloojee 1993b).

Despite the industry's efforts, all of the health groups' recommendations were accepted, with local and national authorities being given the power to restrict smoking in public places and radio commercials again being included in the definition of "advertisements." (In certain cases, however, radio stations could apply for exemption from the requirement to air a health warning as part of tobacco advertisements.) The bill also outlawed the sale of cigarettes to minors and empowered the minister to prescribe the health warning and the details about dangerous ingredients that were to appear on cigarette packs or in advertisements.

Satisfaction Comes with Success

On June 17, 1993, the Tobacco Products Control Act was approved by Parliament. In Venter's own words, she had "ultimately succeeded in arriving at a piece of legislation" that gave her "the most satisfaction of any legislation" since she had had "the privilege of being a minister." Venter made it clear that her business was health and not "problems regarding the cultivation of tobacco." She refrained from becoming involved in or being drawn into a discussion on the interests of tobacco producers, saying, "I really do not believe that it is a matter in which a minister of national health should participate." She also mentioned—tellingly—that she had reconciled herself "long ago that it would not be possible to take everyone along with me and to receive everyone's support for this bill. . . . There are too many vested interests that have to be taken into consideration" (*Hansard* 1993).

Measured against the international "gold standard" for tobacco control legislation, the act was mild. (For legislative "good practice," see PAHO 2002.) However, it "represented a schism between the ruling National Party government and the industry" (van Walbeek 2002a) and was the first major dent in what had been a solid wall of vested interest (Saloojee 1993a). As it turned out, it was the last piece of legislation passed by the National Party government.

New Government, New Regulations

In April 1994 South Africa's first democratic elections were held. The ANC replaced the National Party as the ruling party. Under the new health minister, Nkosazana Zuma, the draft regulations for mandatory and explicit health warnings were published in the *Gazette* for comment. The regulations specified the size of health warnings required on printed advertisements and televised commercials, as well as on cigarette packs. The Health Ministry stated that tobacco industry–sponsored events would not be affected by the directives, as they were examples of "indirect advertising" (Miller and Ramsay 1994). This loophole in the legislation was subsequently exploited by the industry.

Eleven different health warnings, each consisting of two parts, were listed in the regulations (Louw 1994). The first part was a concise warning on the effects of smoking—for example, "Danger, smoking can kill you," and "Pregnant? Breastfeeding? Your smoking could harm your baby." The second part explained how and why smoking damaged health, described the benefits of quitting, and gave a telephone number that smokers who wanted to quit could call to get information and advice. (For example, "Nine out of ten patients with lung cancer are smokers. Smoking also causes cancer of the lip, mouth, voice box, food pipe and bladder. Quitting smoking reduces your risk of cancer. For more information or help call. . . .") Written advertisements only had to carry the first part of the warning, positioned at the top of the advertisement and occupying 10 percent of the area of the advertisement. Another 2 percent of the area had to be dedicated to information on tar and nicotine. Cigarette packs had to carry the two-part warning, which was to occupy 15 percent of the front of the pack and 25 percent of the back.

Antitobacco lobbyists wanted the new labeling in order to give consumers better information about the health hazards of smoking tobacco products, but the cigarette, advertising, and media industries objected strongly (Leaver 2002). TISA sent a submission to the government in which it argued that the regulatory health warnings were unconstitutional because they deprived manufacturers of constitutionally protected property rights of registered trademarks. The industry also asserted that the warnings violated the companies' right to freedom of expression by "compelling manufacturers to include health messages and warnings with a propagandistic character . . . without stating the source" (Leaver 2002). This argument was supported by advertisers, who said that messages without sources gave the "untenable impression that the tobacco advertiser is warning consumers not to use his product" (*Financial Mail* 1994).

Advertisers also claimed that there had been a lack of transparency and consultation in drawing up the draft regulations and that if the regulations became law, there would be numerous job losses in the advertising industry because the tobacco industry would end many of its contracts. The managing director of Times Media Limited, one of South Africa's leading newspaper groups, described the proposals as a form of censorship that trampled on the right to free commercial speech (de Villiers 1994a).

Several newspapers and magazines argued that they stood to lose advertising revenue. The media's opposition was (over)stated in such melodramatic terms as to be almost farcical: the director of Nasionale Pers, in which Rembrandt had shares, predicted a "blood bath" (de Villiers 1994a) and foresaw that the print media would lose millions in revenue and be "paralyzed" (Leaver 2002). The Medical Research Council refuted these absurd claims, quoting a study by the council which had found that in the "10 most popular South African magazines, each with a circulation of over 100,000, tobacco accounted for less than 10% of total adspend" (Leaver 2002).

The one significant concession was that in August 1994 the health minister exempted radio stations from the advertising regulations for one year. Radio stations had argued that they would be hard hit by the new regulations and could lose millions in tobacco advertising revenues (de Villiers 1994a, 1994b). They said they needed time to adjust, since a sudden drop in their revenues might force them to close down broadcasts to isolated and illiterate rural groups, for whom they were a vital source of information and entertainment. For their part, the Independent Broadcasters Association agreed that "the proceeds of five advertising spots per day per radio station which carries tobacco adverts be given to the [health department] for running a campaign aimed at warning people about the dangers of smoking" (de Villiers 1994a, 1994b).

Four months later, in December 1994, the regulations governing the display of health warnings on tobacco products and in advertisements were published in the *Gazette* under the Tobacco Products Control Act of 1993. Enforcement would begin only after several months, to give the tobacco industry time to use up stocks of existing packaging materials. After the legislation was "gazetted," TISA complained that it had not been consulted (Leaver 2002). It had, in fact, voiced its views on several occasions but had not prevailed against the counterarguments and factual evidence presented by the public health groups, which argued that the measures were important for protecting and promoting public health and that the actual economic losses would be trifling, in contrast to the exaggerated claims of those seeking to protect their vested interests.

Implications for the Provinces: New Hope for Cape Town

The implementation of the Tobacco Products Control Act in 1994 was a significant development for municipalities because it granted them the right to apply to the health department to promulgate their own regulations controlling smoking. This was particularly good news for Cape Town because it meant that the administrator no longer had veto power over antismoking measures in the city.

Michael Popkiss, Cape Town's chief medical officer, was quick to apply for these powers. Within four months the Cape Town City Council had tabled draft regulations to restrict smoking in virtually all public places. Specifically, the municipal regulations prohibited smoking in 80 percent of every city restaurant and banned smoking in shopping malls, theaters, cinemas, and all municipal buildings. Public transport, such as trains, buses, and taxis, was also out of bounds for smoking (Oliver 1994). A further stipulation was that any room in which smoking was banned could be designated as a smoking area, provided that a ventilation system was installed to extract the smoky air. The smoking area was not allowed to exceed 20 percent of the total floor area of the enclosed public space, and it had to be clearly signposted.

On March 30, 1995, the antismoking regulations were passed by a large majority of Cape Town's new democratically elected council. A month later, the regulations were published in the *Gazette,* and by August 1995 admission-of-guilt fines for failing to abide by the regulations had been announced by the chief magistrate. The regulations came into full effect on April 26, 1996.

The *Cape Times,* a regional newspaper, was highly critical of the new local legislation, calling it a "gross interference in the free market economy." The newspaper argued that the council should reconsider its decision, as it had no right to tell "private institutions which rely on public patronage for their business what they should, and should not, allow on their property" (*Cape Times* 1995a). This tone was repeated four days later when a *Cape Times* column lent implicit support to restaurant owners who defied the ban. The newspaper published a photograph of the chairman of the Restaurant Guild with a lit cigarette in one hand and a fork in the other, accompanied by a statement describing the new law as "no less ludicrous or impractical than decreeing that 20% of all restaurant windows must be tinted, or that 80% of all tablecloths must be pink" (Jackman 1995).

Many *Cape Times* readers were angered, accusing the newspaper of irresponsible journalism and of supporting the tobacco lobby. Popkiss wrote an open letter in defense of the regulations, noting that their aim was to protect the public from being exposed to the dangers of environmental tobacco smoke and that the council therefore included "any indoor area which is open to the public or any part of the public" in the legislation, regardless of whether it was state owned or privately owned (Popkiss 1995).

Aside from the restaurateurs and some media, negative feedback was limited (Parker 1995). The designers of the new regulations noted that where similar smoking bans existed abroad, the incidence of smoking had decreased because of social pressure rather than the threat of sanctions. Various organizations publicly highlighted their commitment to the new regulations. For example, one of Cape Town's major shopping centers, the Victoria & Alfred Waterfront, voluntarily began a program of educating tenants and staff about the new smoking measures and how best to implement them. Information tables were set up around the shopping center to promote public awareness of the regulations, and bins were placed at mall entrances to allow people to extinguish their cigarettes before entering (Smith 1995). The Cape Town City Council issued a booklet containing details about the legislation and information about the health hazards of smoking, with the aim of educating the public and easing the implementation process.

In October 1995 the Restaurant Guild launched the "Courtesy of Choice" program in an attempt to preempt similar legislation in other provinces. It encouraged South African restaurants to voluntarily cater to both smokers and nonsmokers by giving patrons the option of deciding whether they would like to be seated in a smoking or nonsmoking area (Leaver 2002). The key to the success of the program would be the installation of adequate ventilation in the smoking sections of restaurants. Participating restaurants were given a ventilation checklist, a training video for staff, and a Courtesy of Choice logo, which displayed the message "Welcome smokers and nonsmokers" along with a yin-yang symbol with one half blank and the other half displaying a cigarette.

The NCAS was extremely scornful of the campaign. Saloojee noted that "if common courtesy alone were sufficient to prevent harm, no laws would be needed at all" and that the Restaurant Guild "was disregarding the preferences of nonsmokers, who had stated in surveys that they preferred smoke-free public places" (Strachan 1995).

Almost two years later, in March 1997, an issue of the hospitality industry magazine *Hotel and Caterer* declared that "the fuss created over the past couple of years about cigarette smoking in restaurants seems to have died down." This was attributed directly to the success of the industry's Courtesy of Choice program in fighting "the fanatical antismoking lobby" (Leaver 2002). Little did the restaurant industry know how wrong that analysis was and what was in store.

National Developments

South Africa's tobacco control cause was helped enormously by the first democratic elections in 1994. The new ruling party, the ANC, had no alliance with the tobacco industry and had a much stronger focus on primary health care than the previous government, including a commitment to an effective tobacco control policy.

More than that, Nelson Mandela, the country's new president, had consistently voiced his strong support for antismoking legislation, and he was on record as having called for a "world free of tobacco" (*Republikein* 1994). Mandela's choice for health minister, Nkosazana Zuma, was known to be strong willed and determined. As a physician and asthma sufferer, she was acutely aware of the dangers of passive smoking. A month after taking office, she insisted on smoke-free cabinet meetings, explaining that exposure to tobacco smoke worsened her condition (*Republikein* 1994). Although the tobacco industry had previously been able to delay impending legislation, they were not able to do so with Zuma as health minister. In fact, Zuma often worked at such a pace as to catch the industry off guard, leading to accusations that she was "bulldozing" health bills through Parliament (Stuart 1998).

From the outset, Zuma made it clear that she was going to do everything in her power to reduce tobacco consumption, warning that additional "national legislation would have to be passed if companies did not voluntarily introduce the necessary anti-smoking policies" (Leaver 2002). Saloojee recalled an encounter with Zuma in Harare in November 1993, shortly before she became health minister. Both were attending the historic All Africa Conference on Tobacco and Health.

> Dr Zuma addressed the meeting. . . . She promised that the ANC would ban tobacco advertising, would significantly increase excise taxes, and would regulate tobacco closely. I was sitting next to Dr Zuma. When she returned to her seat, I told her that I had noted everything she had just said and would be holding her to it once she became the health minister. Two months after her appointment, I wrote asking for a meeting. When I entered her office for the meeting, to my amazement, she remembered our conversation and asked: "What took you so long? I've been waiting for you." (Saloojee 2002)

Many prominent delegates to the Harare conference continued on to South Africa afterward, giving major speeches "that helped boost the tobacco control community in the country significantly" (Yach 2002).

Applying Tax Increases

Tobacco lobbyists had long been calling for an increase in taxes on cigarettes. International studies had shown that price was an important determinant of tobacco demand and that raising the price was the single most cost-effective way of quickly reducing consumption. Higher taxes therefore had great potential as a deterrent to smoking. In addition, a tax increase would create more revenue for the government. The NCAS pointed out that because excise taxes had failed to keep up with inflation, the real (inflation-adjusted) tax on cigarettes had fallen by 70 percent between 1970 and 1990 (figure 6.2). Their pleas seemed to have been answered when ANC health advisers proposed a 100 percent increase in cigarette taxes shortly before the 1994 budget. It was a bitter disappointment when finance minister Derek Keys announced a mere 25 percent increase. Antismoking advocates saw the new tax levels as a betrayal of health interests and argued that the budget had effectively sacrificed the lives of thousands of smokers and lost the government millions in revenue. The finance minister responded by saying that as a result of health considerations, the government had agreed to eventually increase the tobacco tax to 50 percent of the retail price of cigarettes. It had opted, however, to phase in the increase; hence the modest rise announced in the current budget.

While tobacco control groups complained that the tax increases were too small, the tobacco industry argued that the hikes were excessive and

Figure 6.2. Real and Nominal Cigarette Prices and Taxes, South Africa, 1961–2000

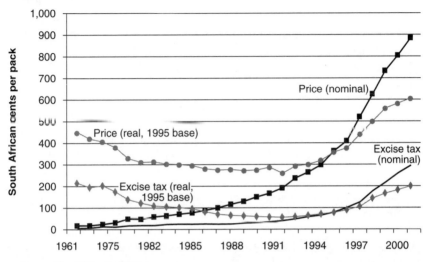

Source: Van Walbeek (2002a).

discriminatory. Rembrandt alleged that smuggled cigarette brands had already started entering South Africa as a result of the new "sin taxes" on tobacco (*Citizen* 1994). The company's new chair, Johann Rupert (Anton Rupert's son) claimed that smuggled brands were undercutting local ones and that this could backfire on the government by negatively affecting state revenues (Leaver 2002). According to van Walbeek (2002a), Rupert's claims were misleading, and deliberately so: if he could persuade the government that cigarette smuggling was increasing as a result of the high taxes, he might also persuade it that the solution would be to reduce the tax.

Only in 1997 was one of the groups finally satisfied, when the new finance minister, Trevor Manuel, announced a tax rate of 50 percent of the retail selling price of cigarettes, after intensive lobbying by Zuma and antismoking groups. Saloojee asserted that the increase would result in 400,000 fewer smokers and an extra 620 million rand in new revenue for the government, which "could be used to employ more customs and excise officials and tighten border controls" (cited in Singh 1997). The tobacco industry was infuriated by the increase, arguing that thousands of the country's farmworkers would lose their jobs. Economists at the University of Cape Town challenged this assertion, pointing out that new jobs would be created to satisfy increased demand for other goods and services as people switched their expenditures from cigarettes to other items. Manuel has since then held firm to his policy and has maintained annual tobacco tax increases of about 50 percent in his budgets (van Walbeek 2002b).

The Struggle for Compliance

In a parliamentary address in October 1996, Zuma accused tobacco companies of ignoring laws requiring the display of health warnings on cigarette packs. The minister warned that "if cigarette companies continued to refuse to comply with the law, her department would respond by banning tobacco advertising" (Leaver 2002). Johann Rupert responded by publishing a full-page open letter to Zuma in the Sunday newspapers saying that the absence of health warnings on certain brands could be blamed on cheaper smuggled goods which had entered South Africa illegally. He alleged that this was the consequence of high tobacco taxes that his company had warned the minister about. In a statement in reply to Rupert's open letter, the minister vowed to intensify her campaign against tobacco, saying, "Responding to individuals is not really our priority at this stage. We are more concerned with the health of the nation" (Leaver 2002).

Meanwhile, cigarette companies and broadcasters took advantage of a loophole in the advertising restrictions in the Tobacco Products Control Act. The act considered sports sponsorships an indirect form of advertising, thus exempting such events from having to display health warnings. The SABC showed Benson & Hedges logos on television during an international cricket match, maintaining that displaying a logo, however prominent, did not constitute advertising (Rulashe 1996). Both the SABC and the tobacco company were strongly criticized, and Zuma threatened to take serious action against companies that were considering "taking advantage of loopholes" in the future (Leaver 2002; see also figure 6.3).

The minister's unwavering political support for tobacco control and her outspoken behavior left her rather exposed. The tobacco industry spent sizable amounts on generating research supporting its position or trying to cast doubts on the arguments and evidence put forward by the public health groups (Wilkins 2000). Clearly, the industry could outspend the groups that were lobbying for tobacco control.

In 1996 an important new partner joined the tobacco control lobby when a number of professional economists entered the debate and set up the Economics of Tobacco Control in South Africa (ETCSA) Project. The project, established at the Applied Fiscal Research Centre of the University of Cape Town with funding from the International Tobacco Initiative (now Research for International Tobacco Control, a secretariat at the International Development Research Centre in Canada), aimed to make

Figure 6.3. Zuma versus Rupert: A Cartoonist's View

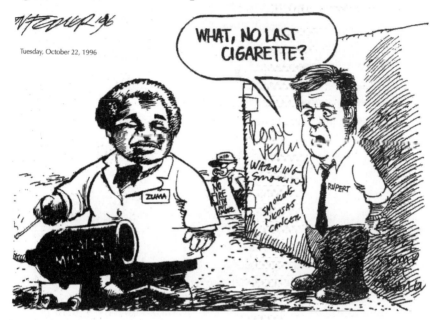

Tuesday, October 22, 1996

Health Minister Zuma prepares to obliterate tobacco company chair Rupert's opposition to tobacco control. The "writing on the wall" is a set of antismoking statements. *Source: The Star,* October 22, 1996.

available to the government and to others sound and accessible information on tobacco control by systematically researching economic issues and providing facts that contradicted the false claims of the tobacco lobby (Abedian 2002).

The ETCSA Project's research findings countered many of the industry's claims and were well publicized. According to Iraj Abedian, ETCSA's project leader at the time, the findings provided important evidence to support Zuma's anti-tobacco policies and the tax increases. One of the most significant conclusions was that a rise in tobacco excise taxes would increase government revenues, not reduce total revenues as the tobacco lobby claimed. In fact, the research demonstrated that the government was earning much less than it could from tobacco taxes: it was estimated that had the state attempted to maximize its revenue from cigarettes, excise receipts could have been 129 percent higher in 1995 than they actually were (see figure 6.4). Other findings were that job losses in tobacco-related sectors would be more than compensated for by job gains in other sectors, since consumers would spend their money on other

Figure 6.4. Potential and Actual Cigarette Tax Revenues (Excise and Sales Taxes Combined), South Africa, 1971–2000

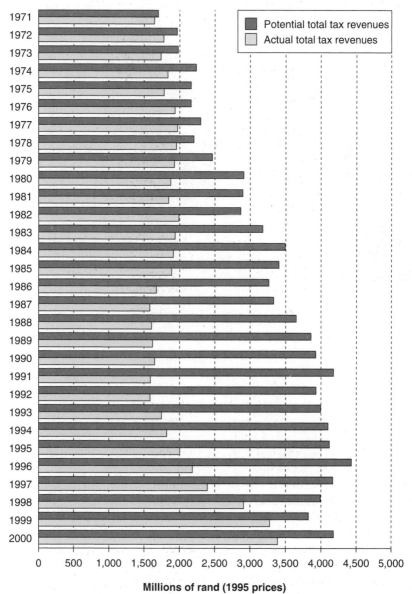

Source: Van Walbeek (2002a).

goods and services, and that South Africa did not have a significant cigarette smuggling problem (van Walbeek 2002a).

Evidence that the government's tobacco control policy was proving effective emerged in May 1996, when a survey found that the proportion of adults who were currently smokers had declined from 34 percent in February 1995 to 32 percent a year later. It also revealed that more than 8 out of 10 adults viewed health warnings on cigarette packs as helpful and informative. These findings convinced the health minister "that mandatory health warnings on tobacco packaging had proven to be an effective tool in educating the public about the dangers of smoking" (Leaver 2002). An anecdote illustrates the power of these warnings for certain consumers: some shopkeepers reported that shortly after the warnings were introduced, some customers asked for the "old" cigarettes rather than the "new" ones, pointing to the warnings and saying that the new ones would cause them to get sick. These customers assumed that the product had changed, necessitating the new warnings (Saloojee 2002).

Within a year after taking office, Nelson Mandela was awarded two no-smoking medals: one in August 1994 by the Commonwealth Games Council and another in May 1995 by the World Health Organization (WHO). On accepting the latter award on his behalf in Vancouver, Canada, Minister of Health Zuma said that millions of children faced premature death from diseases caused by tobacco, and that "this preventable tragedy must be averted" (Strachan 1995).

1999 Legislation

In January 1998 the health minister announced that a Tobacco Control Amendment Bill would be tabled in Parliament that year. Initially, Zuma gave little indication of precisely what changes it would entail. Addressing a tobacco conference in February, however, she hinted at "an outright ban on advertising, sponsorships and promotions, and raising the age at which minors could legally buy cigarettes to 18" (Leaver 2002).

Six months after the minister had announced her plans, the Tobacco Products Control Amendment Bill was unanimously approved by the cabinet. Among other provisions, it outlawed smoking in enclosed public spaces (including workplaces), banned tobacco advertising and sponsorship, and made it illegal for anyone to sell cigarettes without the prescribed health warnings on packs (Soal 1998a).

The cigarette manufacturing industry slammed the health department for tabling a "draconian bill out of the blue eight weeks before Parliament closes" (Leaver 2002). Many opposition parties agreed, remarking that "the Zuma Bulldozer is clearly in overdrive" (Stuart 1998). The industry complained that the tobacco control lobby had benefited from many months of access during the bill's drafting process, whereas the tobacco industry had been totally excluded from the process. Cigarette companies, along with advertising and freedom of expression organizations, argued that the legislation was a gross violation of the right to freedom of speech. But Zuma had no interest in modifying the proposals in response to pressure from the industry, and she threatened to take the battle to the country's highest court (Khan 1998).

Zuma even went a step further: when President Mandela asked her to consult with all relevant parties before pressing ahead, she called them together on short notice late one night. Also at the meeting were tobacco control advocates, including the Medical Research Council's Derek Yach. Yach had to counter the fears of the media companies that they would lose a large part of their income because of the ban on tobacco advertising. When he reminded them that "it's better to associate with life than with death," one of the country's largest publishing houses, Caxton, which published many medical publications and also community newspapers, voluntarily withdrew its tobacco advertising in advance of the law (Yach 2002).

Pro-tobacco groups had the opportunity to present arguments as well. Yach recalled that a tobacco representative asked Zuma toward the end of the meeting whether she had listened to their arguments and whether she was going to weaken the legislation as a result. She responded, "If anything I'll consider strengthening it, because I don't believe what you're saying" (Yach 2002).

Sporting organizations did not feel comfortable with the bill, as they stood to lose sponsorship from cigarette companies. The South African tobacco industry annually spent about 40 million rand on sports events such as Winfield rugby, the Rothmans July Handicap, the Gunston 500 (an international surfing competition), and Rothmans soccer. The Premier Soccer League was particularly concerned, as it had a 10-year contract with Rothmans worth 100 million rand that it believed would be difficult to replace (Khan 1998).

Zuma's proposals also ended South Africa's Grand Prix hopes. Earlier that year the chief executive of Formula One Grand Prix had announced that South Africa was being considered as a possible host in the near future. But with the tobacco industry being the main motor racing sponsor and competitors contractually obliged to carry their sponsors' names on their cars, the event would not be allowed in South Africa under the proposed legislation. Shortly after the bill was tabled, Formula One released its race calendar, and South Africa was notably absent. Malaysia, a country with no restrictions on tobacco advertising, had taken its place.

Zuma responded to these concerns by noting that cricket had cut its ties with its tobacco sponsor (Benson & Hedges) some time earlier and that the sport continued to prosper. The tobacco control proponents also pointed out that tobacco-sponsored events were a betrayal of the millions of youths who looked to sports to promote health, not to promote a deadly addiction (Saloojee 2002). In an attempt to alleviate some of the fears, Zuma and the sports minister discussed plans to phase in the restrictions in order to protect existing sponsorships. Ever determined, however, Zuma commented that "it will be a very short phase-in. If they have a 10-year contract, they won't be able to finish it" (Soal 1998b).

Two weeks after being approved by the cabinet, the Tobacco Products Amendment Bill was published for public comment. Twelve days later, the tobacco industry applied for an urgent interdict to stall the legislation, citing "a lack of consultation in the bill's drafting" (Leaver 2002). Zuma was undeterred and told a journalist that "consultation does not mean we must keep consulting with them until they agree" and that she was now "more than ever determined to get the legislation through Parliament" (Soal 1998b). The applicants asked the Cape Town High Court to order the minister to disclose "all the information that the department had taken into account when drafting the bill" (Leaver 2002). But the case was dismissed eight days later; the court ruled that the information was public knowledge, and Zuma proclaimed that no one would be allowed to filibuster the process (Baleta and Oliver 1998).

Two months later, a public hearing, dubbed by some as being like "the biblical battle between David and Goliath," was scheduled in Parliament. More than 80 groups applied to give oral evidence over two days. Three days after the hearings, the parliamentary health committee approved the bill, to the dismay of cigarette companies. Yet again, the tobacco industry threatened to go to court, but, as in the past, the threat failed to materialize. Instead, after a day's heated debate, the National Assembly approved the proposed legislation, with 213 votes (all from the ANC and the African Christian Party) in favor and 106 against.

Following approval by the National Council of Provinces, the bill was sent to the president for his signature. Mandela, however, sent it back to Parliament, asking that the terms "organized activity" and "public places" be more clearly defined to resolve constitutional uncertainties. The president specifically wanted clarity on whether public places included private residences in which employees such as domestic workers performed their duties. Of particular concern was that "people may not be able to smoke in their own homes if they employ a domestic worker," although, on the other hand, domestic workers should not be subjected to the health risk posed by secondhand smoke (Saloojee 1999).

A month later, the health department had completed the work of drafting amendments to the definitions in question, with "public places" cited as including workplaces but not private homes. In March 1999 the amendments were approved by both the National Assembly and the National Council of Provinces. Only two provinces, the Western Cape, held by the National Party, and Kwazulu-Natal, held by the Inkatha Freedom Party, voted against the bill. The Tobacco Products Amendment Act became law on April 23, 1999, when it was published in the *Gazette*. (The legislation would only come into effect once a date had been set by promulgation in the *Gazette*.)

The tobacco control lobby was extremely satisfied with the new legislation, with the Medical Research Council remarking that the act was "a fitting finale to Mandela's term of office because it would entrench laws that will protect children for generations to come" (Leaver 2002). The act came into effect on October 1, 2000, with the new health minister, Dr. Manto Tshabalala-Msimang, saying that she did not expect any constitutional challenges. After January 2001, anyone found guilty of disobeying the law (except for restaurant owners who had applied for a six months' exemption to install nonsmoking areas) would be liable to a fine.

Zuma's tough stance against smoking was recognized by the WHO in May 1999, with the Tobacco Free World Award. The organization's director-general, Gro Harlem Brundtland, told Zuma, "We congratulate you on your work—you have strengthened our hands and given hope to many countries" (WHO 1999).

Back in South Africa, the tobacco and advertising industries continued their exaggerated, even absurd, rhetoric, comparing the new legislation to laws enacted by Nazi Germany and referring to Zuma as a "new Hitler." The minister replied, "I'm getting used to the names by now. What is important is whether we are transforming society for the better, and I think we are" (Soal 1998b).

Conclusion

Derek Yach believes there is an important lesson to be learned from South Africa's achievements: "You need the right combination of science, evidence and politics to succeed. If you have one without the other, you don't see action." He believes that South Africa has had an effective mix of basic science, political commitment, and the ability to move ahead (Yach 2002).

Despite the significant opposition encountered, South Africa now has one of the most comprehensive tobacco control policies in the world. Van Walbeek (2002b) noted that "while the health impact of the change of smoking patterns will only be felt in years to come, the short-term measurable outcomes suggest that the South African government's tobacco control policy is proving successful: between 1993 and 2000, total tobacco consumption decreased by about 26% . . . per capita consumption

Figure 6.5. Real Cigarette Prices and Smoking Prevalence by Income Group, South Africa, 1993–2000

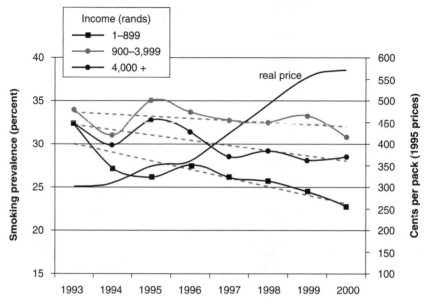

Source: Van Walbeek (2002a).

decreased by 37% . . . the percent of adults who smoke decreased from 33% to 27%, with the biggest decreases being seen in low income groups . . . and the percent of young people aged 16 to 24 who smoke has decreased significantly from 24% to 19%." Figure 6.5 clearly shows the decline in consumption across all income groups and the much faster and deeper decrease in smoking in the lower-income groups.

Although the degree of compliance with antismoking legislation seems to be high, some say more can be done. Saloojee points out that despite significant increases in tobacco taxes, cigarettes in South Africa are still very cheap in comparison with other countries and that they continue to be affordable, particularly for young people. (See figure 3.2, in chapter 3 in this volume, which compares cigarette prices across a number of countries.) He adds that it is almost impossible to institute legal action for medical damages against cigarette companies without having "sizable amounts of money." Saloojee also points out that some countries, such as Canada and Brazil, now require large pictorial warnings on tobacco products—"something which South Africa needs to consider if we want to keep up with leading tobacco control countries in the world" (Saloojee 2002).

References

Abedian, I. 2002. Personal communication, June 3.

Baleta, A., and L. Oliver. 1998. "Zuma Snuffs Giants: Tobacco War Victory." *The Independent on Saturday,* Sept. 5.

Barrett, C. 1989. "Smoke-Free Zones: PE Takes a Stand." *Weekend Post,* Oct. 14.

Bateman, C. 1989a. "Civic Uproar over Smoking: Leading Lights Defend Popkiss." *Argus,* March.

____. 1989b. "City's Smoke Ban Angers Anton Rupert." *Argus,* April.

Burgers, L. 1991. "Clampdown on Puffing in Restaurants." *The Star,* March 27.

Cape Argus. 1988. "Smoking Restricted in City Restaurants, Adverts Banned." March 28.

____. 1989a. "Anton Rupert Sends Retort over No-Smoking Issue." March.

____. 1989b. "Medical Campus Smoking Ban." March.

Cape Times. 1991. "Did Tobacco Chiefs Stub Curbs Plan?" May 7.

____. 1995a. "City Dictatorship on Smoking." April 3.

____. 1995b. "Seven Million Can't Be Extinguished." June 1.

Cape Town Chamber of Commerce. 1990. "Smoking Ban Reversed." *Cape Town Chamber of Commerce Weekly Bulletin,* March.

Chapman, S., D. Yach, Y. Saloojee, and D. Simpson. 1994. "All Africa Conference on Tobacco Control." *British Medical Journal* 308: 189–91.

Citizen. 1994. "High Excise Increases Cigarette Smuggling." July 28.

Dennehy, P. 1989a. "Council Curbs Employees Smoking." *Cape Times,* March 31.

____. 1989b. "City Smoke Ban Vetoed." *Cape Times,* April.

de Villiers, L. 1994a. "Ad Industry Comes out Smoking." *Weekend Star,* Aug. 20–21.

____. 1994b. "SABC Radio Gets Tobacco Reprieve." *The Star,* Aug. 26.

Doman, A. 1989a. "Restaurant Smoking Ban Backed by Health Council." *Argus,* March 30.

____. 1989b. "Restaurateurs Give Council Week to Scrap Ban." *Argus,* July 28.

____. 1989c. "Restaurant Owners to Fight Ban on Smoking." *Argus,* July 27.

East London Daily Dispatch. 1991. "SABC Refuses to Screen Anti-Smoking Advert." May 4.

Financial Mail. 1994. "Putting out Fires." Sept. 2.

Fothergill, M. 1991. "Smoking Comes under Fire." *Business Day,* April 8.

Hansard. 1993. *Debates of Parliament,* no. 19, Republic of South Africa. Fifth Session–Ninth Parliament. June 1–4: 10105–58.

Hotel and Caterer. 1995. "Separate—Then Ventilate!" Nov., 33–37.

Jackman, T. 1995. "Blow Smoke in the Face of Insanity." *Cape Times,* April 7.

Khan, F. 1998. "Smoking Ad Row Flares." *Natal Daily News,* July 31.

Leaver, R. 2002. "Tobacco Control Policy in South Africa as Seen through the Eyes of the Media." In C. van Walbeek, *The Economics of Tobacco Control in South Africa.* University of Cape Town.

Levy, T. 1991a. "Fired-up Ads from the Anti-Smoking Gun." *Business Day,* April 4.

____. 1991b. "Anti-Smoking Ads Banned by SABC TV." *Business Day,* April 5.

Louw, C. 1994. "Warning: The Regulation of Tobacco Ads Can Be Hazardous." *Weekly Mail and Guardian,* July 8.

Medicine Today. 1991. "Smoking Ad Laws Do Not Go Far Enough—MRC." June 27.

Miller, S., and R. Ramsay. 1994. "Smoking Risk Ads Become Law Soon." *Natal Daily News,* June 22.

Morris, M. 1989. "Rupert Warns of 'Mafia' Tobacco Swoop." *Argus,* March 9.

Natal Daily News. 1991. "Local Media Drawn into Anti-Smoking Ads." April.

———. 1995. "No Smoking Ignored." April 3.

Nevill, G., and G. Gill. 1991. "Smoking Ban out of Puff?" *Cape Times,* March 28.

Oliver, L. 1994. "Council to Stub Smoking from Enclosed Public Places." *Argus,* Sept. 7.

PAHO (Pan American Health Organization). 2002. "Developing Legislation for Tobacco Control." Washington, D.C. Available at <www.paho.org/English/HPP/HPM/TOH/tobacco_legislation.htm>.

Parker, W. 1995. "Smokers Meekly Accept Cape Town's Ban." *Business Day,* April 25.

P.E. Advertiser. 1999. "Zuma Gets Tobacco Free World Award." May 18.

Perlman, J. 1991a. "Rina Venter Kicks the Butts." *Weekly Mail,* June 27.

———. 1991b. "Anti-Tobacco Lobby Comes out Smoking as State Stalls." *Weekly Mail,* July 12.

———. 1993. "Better Air or Smoking Ban?" *The Star,* Jan. 30.

Popkiss, M. 1995. "Clearing up the Confusion." *Cape Times,* April 25.

Pretoria News. 1994. "Public Smoke Ban on Cards." May 31.

Republikein. 1994. "SA Government Wants to Avoid Smoking" (in Afrikaans). June 1.

Rulashe, L. 1996. "Plan to Stub out Smoking 'Pimps.'" *Sunday Times,* Jan. 14.

Saloojee, Y. 1993a. "Tobacco Control: A Case Study (South Africa)." In *Proceedings of the All Africa Conference on Tobacco and Health. 1 November 1993, Harare, Zimbabwe.*

———. 1993b. "A Misinformation Industry." *Business Day,* Oct. 29.

———. 1999. Statement on the referral of the tobacco bill to Parliament (news release), Jan. 22. Tobacco Action Group.

———. 2002. Personal communication.

Singh, P. 1997. "Anti-Smokers Warn against Pressure from Tobacco Industry." *The Star,* March 31.

Smith, D. 1995. "Waterfront Joins Battle." *Cape Times,* Oct. 30.

Soal, J. 1998a. "Government's Tough New Curbs on Smoking." *Cape Times,* July 15.

———. 1998b. "Every Which Way, Smokers Are on the Run." *The Star,* Aug. 7.

South African Medical Journal. 1963. "Cigarettes and Smoking" (editorial), 37 (39): 974–75.

Steenkamp, W. 1994. "Tobacco Giants Hit back at 'Total Onslaught' on Ads." *Argus,* June 4.

Strachan, K. 1995. "No-Smoking Bylaw Has Guild Fuming." *Business Day,* Oct. 10.

Stuart, B. 1998. "Zuma Accused of Bulldozing Bills." *Citizen,* Sept. 5.

van Walbeek, C. 2002a. *The Economics of Tobacco Control in South Africa.* University of Cape Town.

———. 2002b. Personal communication, May 17.

Wilkins, N. 2000. "The Economics of Tobacco Control in South Africa: Lessons for Tobacco Control Toolkit Development." March 30–31. Briefing note prepared for the WHO meeting on the Development of Toolkits for Tobacco Control Legislation and Economic Interventions, Geneva.

Woodgate, S. 1991. "Ban Goes up in Puff of Smoke." *The Star*, April 24.

World Health Organization. 1999. Speech by Director-General Gro Harlem Brundtland. Geneva.

Yach, D. 1982. "Economic Aspects of Smoking in South Africa." *South African Medical Journal* 62: 167–70.

———. 2002. Personal communication.

Yach, D., and G. Townsend. 1988. "Smoking and Health in South Africa: The Need for Action." Technical Report 1. April. South African Medical Research Council, Parow.

Yach, D., Y. Saloojee, and D. McIntyre. 1992. "Smoking in South Africa: Health and Economic Impact." South African Medical Research Council, Cape Town.

7

Tailoring Tobacco Control Efforts to the Country: The Example of Thailand

Prakit Vateesatokit

The need for tobacco control in Thailand is evident in the statistics. Among Thailand's 62 million inhabitants, fewer than 5 percent of females smoke, but 39 percent of males do (National Statistics Office 1999). Although the recent economic downturn and increases in cigarette taxes contributed to a decline in consumption from 48 billion cigarettes in 1997 to 37 billion in 2001, the toll from tobacco use is still heavy. It has been estimated that in 1993, 42,000 Thais died of tobacco-attributable disease (Ekplakorn, Wongkraisrithong, and Tangchareonsin 1991). Lung cancer is the number one cancer in Thai males except in the northeastern region, where endemic liver fluke disease makes liver cancer more common (Deerasamee and others 1999).

Understanding Thailand's efforts to work toward successful tobacco control requires an appreciation of the complex sociocultural, political, and even personal dynamics that interact to shape Thai thinking and policymaking. These dynamics cannot be captured in a short case study and are not fully described in this deeply personal account, in which the political, social, and human factors are intimately entwined.

The narrative shows that while similarities exist between the Thai experience and that of other countries, the success of tobacco control in Thailand must also be attributed to a unique historical struggle set in the rich context of Thai politics and culture (Muscat 1992). Furthermore, it is a story grounded in the rational, iterative world of medical investigation and the sometimes chaotic world of political process. Combined, these ingredients make for a fascinating story.

The Story Begins: Small Steps Forward

The best-known incident in tobacco control in Thailand is the well-publicized case in the late 1980s when the U.S. tobacco industry used international trade treaty provisions to force open Asian markets to foreign cigarettes. But the struggle for tobacco control in Thailand began long before that, as early as the mid-1970s. In 1974 the Thai Medical Association successfully petitioned the government to print health warnings on cigarette packages. In 1976 the National Statistics Office carried out the first national survey of smoking prevalence (now conducted every two to three years as part of the National Health and Welfare Survey), and the Bangkok Metropolitan Administration issued an ordinance banning smoking in movie theatres and buses in the city. When the World Health Organization (WHO) designated 1980 the Year of the No Smoking Campaign, the event was supported by the Thai Ministry of Public Health (MOPH), the Thai Thoracic Association, the Thai Anti-Tuberculosis Association, and the Thai Heart Association. A series of public health education programs on the dangers of smoking was carried out, and the Thai Tobacco Monopoly (TTM) was successfully lobbied to strengthen the health warning on cigarette packages.

Other sporadic activities and campaigns were undertaken in the 1980s, with mixed results. In 1982 the MOPH and the WHO held the First National Conference on Tobacco or Health. Subsequently, an expert committee was established to implement an ongoing campaign to reduce smoking, but because there was no secretariat or organizational support, the committee met infrequently, and little was accomplished. The National Cancer Institute listed cigarettes as a cause of cancer and carried out public education seminars. Tobacco was also included as a health issue of the noncommunicable disease division in the MOPH's Department of Medical Services. But without continuous, sustained momentum, these efforts had only limited outcomes (Supawongse 1999). When the Thai Anti-Smoking Campaign Project (TASCP) was formed in 1986, the media commented that they hoped it would not be just another "flash in the pan" that would die away (TASCP 1986).

In a parallel development, in the 1980s health professionals, perceiving a need to improve the level of health advocacy in the country, established the Folk Doctors Foundation (FDF). The FDF focused on self-care, used public advocacy, and disseminated information through educational materials and the media to foster a social movement supporting care for the health of the Thai population. These efforts were early examples of the potential role of a nongovernmental organization (NGO) in tobacco control.

In early 1986 Dr. Pravase Wasi, an FDF board member, respected university professor, and opinion leader, gave a presentation to the Dusit Rotary Club on tobacco and health. This presentation resulted in a contribution of 60,000 baht (US$2,255) for tobacco control efforts. Initially, Wasi had intended to give the money to those in the MOPH who were working on tobacco control. At the time, however, no special office existed for this type of activity, so he decided it would be more efficient to turn the money over to the FDF to support a specific project on tobacco control.

With this fund, in October 1986 Wasi launched the TASCP at Ramathibodi Hospital, along with another FDF board member, Prof. Athasit Vejjajiva, who had just become dean at Ramathibodi Hospital, Faculty of Medicine, Mahidol University. Dr. Paibul Suriyawongpaisal of the Department of Community Medicine was appointed secretary of the project. The author, who was the chairman of the Department of Medicine, was asked to take part in the launch by helping to organize a press conference on the harm caused by tobacco use. Four patients with chronic obstructive lung disease were asked to speak about their suffering, showing the "human face" of the epidemic. This proved very successful in attracting press coverage.

As a result, the author was recruited to join the TASCP, which would serve as a focal point and pressure group in the lobby for tobacco control policy. One of the first tasks was to work with Dr. Somkiat Onvimol and Laddawan Wongsriwong to produce a three-minute spot documenting the life of a patient who suffered from emphysema and was receiving home oxygen therapy. This documentary was aired several times in 1987 and inspired several young doctors from another NGO, the Rural Doctors' Association (RDA), to organize a run in support of the antismoking cause. Dr. Choochai Supawongse, RDA chair, first developed the idea of the nationwide run with support from the MOPH and other funding organizations. The 250 physicians and paramedics who participated ran a total of over 3,000 kilometers in the span of a week. The campaign collected over 6 million signatures of townspeople along the way, all urging Parliament to legislate tobacco control.

The organized run was another example of sporadic, uncoordinated, but genuine and sometimes dramatic efforts by various professional groups that arose out of their personal commitment to reducing harm from tobacco. Many doctors who are now senior officials trace their strong commitment to tobacco control to this event (Supawongse 1999).

Building Support: The TASCP's Formative Years

Those working for tobacco control in the early years did not fully appreciate the importance of having a comprehensive and coherent strategy until 1987, when the Sixth World Conference on Tobacco or Health was held in Japan. That conference was an eye-opener and provided additional impetus to the TASCP. Dr. Halfdan Mahler, then director general of the WHO, delivered a provocative speech about smoking mortality, describing it as equivalent to 20 jumbo jets crashing each day, or 2 million deaths per year. The diversity of the audience of epidemiologists, public health workers, activists, and media advocates reflected the broad implications of the issue. It became clear at the conference that the epidemic would not disappear soon or on its own: a policy response was essential.

As a direct result of the conference, the TASCP developed its first educational poster. At the conference, Dr. Jureerut Bornvornwattanuvongs, a pulmonary disease specialist at Chonburi provincial hospital, presented a research paper reporting smoking rates for doctors, teachers, and Buddhist monks—all influential opinion leaders in Thai society. The TASCP used this research information to focus on a campaign to change the regular practice of offering cigarettes to monks. Posters reading "Offering cigarettes to monks is a sin" were printed and distributed, as well as "Smoke-free zone" and "Thank you for not smoking" stickers. The TASCP's approach was to remain positive—not to condemn smokers, but to oppose pushing cigarettes on others.

Subsequently, in 1988, the TASCP took advantage of a clinical epidemiology conference in Thailand, where Dr. Richard Peto, an epidemiologist and statistician from Oxford University, was the featured speaker. Peto later proved to be a very helpful resource in Thailand's tobacco control struggle. The TASCP used the opportunity of the conference to call for action to prevent 1 million Thai children from dying from cigarette smoking, as had been projected by Peto (TASCP 1988).

All of these efforts and early successes set the stage for Thailand's later determination to fight the U.S. trade sanctions.

Challenges from Beyond: Tobacco Trade Wars

In the late 1980s Thailand was suddenly awash with cigarette advertisements. The Thai Tobacco Monopoly (TTM) began promoting its product in response to the sudden appearance of advertisements for foreign cigarette brands. Until then, the TTM had seen no reason to advertise, since it was a monopoly and foreign cigarette brands were available only illegally or through airport duty-free shops in Bangkok. In the words of the U.S. Tobacco Merchants Association, the Thai state-run tobacco industry, which had come into existence to displace British American Tobacco after World War II, was "fat and extremely uncompetitive" (Tobacco Merchants Association 1988). But now the TTM faced an advertising war with foreign producers (Frankel 1996). Meanwhile, the TASCP, concerned that the foreign companies were advertising in an effort to launch their brands in Thailand, urged the government to ban all advertising, both domestic and foreign.

In January 1988 the TTM applied to the cabinet for funds to build a new, more productive, and more efficient tobacco factory. Although the project was initially approved, the decision was soon reversed because of media protests fueled by the TASCP. General Prem—a respected career soldier who was invited to be prime minister for eight years by the elected coalition parties, even though he had not run for election—was responsive to tobacco control advocates. He said at the time that it was not right for the government to obtain income from such an inappropriate source. He did allocate some funds for new machinery for the TTM's existing factory, but at the same time the cabinet instructed the MOPH to draft a plan for tobacco control.

In April 1988 the MOPH presented a tobacco control plan that was approved by the cabinet in its entirety. Dr. Hatal Chitanondh, deputy director general of the ministry's Department of Medical Services, was responsible for drafting the comprehensive plan. One of the components was an advertising ban, which the TTM did not object to, since it knew it could never match the huge resources of the international tobacco companies.

In December 1988, however, when the international tobacco companies were still advertising (claiming that the prohibition by the cabinet was an executive order, not a law, and therefore did not have to be followed by the private sector), the TTM protested to the government. The cabinet directed the Consumer Protection Board, a government agency operating under the auspices of the Prime Minister's Office, to find a means of stopping cigarette advertising by law. In February 1989 the board added tobacco to the list of regulated products that could not be advertised under the 1979 Consumer Protection Act. The international companies were given one month to dismantle and remove all their billboards and advertisements. (They refused to comply for nine months.)

In February 1989 the cabinet appointed the National Committee for the Control of Tobacco Use (NCCTU), as specified in the tobacco control plan. The committee was chaired by Chuan Leekpai, minister of public health, and included members from the TASCP and the press. Chitanondh served as secretary. It was clear then that the committee would have to formulate and coordinate a comprehensive tobacco control policy.

In March 1989, when the Ministry of Finance proposed opening the market to foreign cigarettes, the author, as the TASCP's executive secretary, personally handed a letter to Major General Chunhawan, the new prime minister, opposing the move. The NCCTU followed up with another letter to the cabinet. In response, the ministry withdrew the market-opening proposal, and the matter was believed to be settled. It came as a shock when, only two months later, it was learned that the U.S. Trade Office had accepted the U.S. Cigarette Export Association's petition to investigate Thailand under Section 301 of the 1974 U.S. Trade Act. No one had thought that Thailand could be forced to open the market (Vateesatokit 1996), and the strength of the U.S. tobacco lobby had certainly been underestimated.

Minister of Public Health Leekpai immediately expressed his opposition to the U.S. use of the Trade Act against Thailand, and within a month international support was growing for the country's stand. In June the John Tung Foundation, an NGO in Taipei, Taiwan (China), that concentrates on tobacco control, invited the author to represent Thailand at a meeting to discuss, plan, and lay out a strategy. The foundation feared that Thailand was just a step toward opening the whole Asian market. About two dozen people attended the conference. Among them were Ted Chen, representing the American Public Health Association, Greg Connolly from the Massachusetts Department of Health, Richard Daynard from Northeastern University in Boston, and Terry Pechacek from the U.S. National Cancer Institute. Others at the meeting included tobacco control advocates from Japan, the Republic of Korea, and Taiwan (China), all of which had reluctantly given in to U.S. pressure on cigarette trade under Section 301. It was hoped that Thailand would take a strong stand and avoid the same problem. At the conclusion of the meeting, the Asia-Pacific Association for the Control of Tobacco (APACT) was established. The conference resolution called for U.S. president George H. W. Bush to exclude tobacco from the Section 301 trade items and for APACT to coordinate tobacco control activities in the region. Thailand would be the test case (Chen and Elaimy 1994).

Point–Counterpoint: Trade versus Health

At the APACT meeting, Connolly strongly suggested negotiating the tobacco control issue with the U.S. Trade Office from the perspective of health rather than trade. Initially Thailand had no health representative in its delegation, and there was some resistance to the author's participation for fear of irritating the Trade Office. The author did manage to work himself onto the delegation and, along with Dr. Surin Pitsuwan, a Harvard-educated Democrat member of Parliament, asked for a public hearing to present Thailand's case. The two also lobbied health organizations and made presentations at international conferences describing the threat to Thailand.

In a short space of time in 1990 the author attended several complementary events to gain support for Thailand. First was the American Cancer Society's "Trade for Life Campaign" summit in Washington, D.C., attended by world tobacco control leaders, where the GLOBALink computer network to speed tobacco control communications was launched. Next was the Seventh World Conference on Tobacco or Health, in Perth, Australia. There Connolly and the author worked on strategies for negotiations with the U.S. Trade Office and for the U.S. congressional hearings scheduled for May (Vateesatokit 1990b). Along with William Foege, who was then executive director of the Carter Center, they testified before the U.S. Senate Committee on Labor and Human Resources, chaired by Sen. Edward Kennedy.[1] Following that, Dr. Judith Mackay of the Asian Tobacco Consultancy, John Seffrin of the American Cancer Society, Carlos Alvarez Herrera, from Argentina and chairman of the Latin American Coordinating Committee on Smoking and Health, and the author testified before the House Committee on Energy and Commerce, Subcommittee on Health and the Environment, chaired by Rep. Henry Waxman. At the 15th International Cancer Conference, held in August 1990 in Hamburg, Germany, with support from the American Cancer Society, the author presented the Thai case in a last effort to build support (Vateesatokit 1990a).

After two inconclusive rounds of negotiations with the Thai government, the U.S. Trade Office referred the dispute to a General Agreement on Tariffs and Trade (GATT) panel. Several rounds of testimony before the panel were held in 1990, with the WHO supporting Thailand and the European Union supporting the United States. Finally, the GATT ruled that Thailand's import ban was contrary to trade provisions but that Thailand could maintain and introduce tobacco control measures as long as they applied to both domestic and foreign products (GATT 1990; for the details of the GATT adjudication, see Chitanondh 2001).

Toward the end, when the GATT decision was known but not yet announced, the U.S. Trade Office made one last unsuccessful attempt to gain victory by obtaining Thailand's signature on an agreement that would have allowed point-of-sale promotion—something that is prohibited under Thailand's tobacco control law of 1989. The Thai cabinet moved quickly to declare the market open and notified the U.S. Trade Office that they had done so, thus precluding any further negotiations or the need to sign any agreements. With that, the dispute with the U.S. Trade Office was over—but the struggle with the international tobacco companies had barely begun.

The Section 301 trade dispute occurred under General Chunhawan's coalition government. Although the Chart Thai Party was the core of the government, Chuan Leekpai's Democrat Party played a major role. Leekpai, who was then deputy prime minister, is an honest, respected politician with close links to the TASCP. In the coalition government, Leekpai's party was in charge of the MOPH and took a strong stand in the negotiations with the U.S. Trade Office, arguing the health and moral aspects of tobacco trade. The prolonged negotiations provided considerable opportunities for antismoking advocates to keep the issue before the public.

---

1. The Carter Center is an NGO based in Atlanta, Ga., and headed by former U.S. president Jimmy Carter. It is active on a number of international issues.

This enhanced the advocates' bargaining power and ensured the account-ability of the government (Chitanondh 2001).

The Ministry of Finance adopted a low-key approach in the tobacco policy debate, primarily providing information on the TTM's operations. Although the Trade Ministry was the accused party in the dispute, it let the health representatives argue Thailand's case for the import ban. In response to the U.S. complaint to the GATT regarding a discriminatory internal excise tax, the tax was adjusted to a single flat rate. The Trade Ministry acknowledged early on that smoking is hazardous to health and did not oppose the Consumer Protection Board's new regulation for warning labels on the front of cigarette packs; thus, it showed that it would comply with the government's tobacco control policy.

By contrast, the Ministry of Commerce was initially uncomfortable with the role of health groups in the negotiating process. As head of the negotiating team, the Commerce Ministry was keenly aware of the many other trade issues at stake and feared that the MOPH representatives would take an uncompromising stand that could lead to trade retaliation. After a few rounds of talks, however, the ministry began to see the impor-tance of using health issues to argue the case and agreed to include MOPH representatives (Hatai Chitanondh and the author) in its official delegation when the case went to the GATT. Meanwhile, the U.S. Trade Office continued to insist that the issue was one of trade only, and it did not include a health representative in its delegation.

The Ministry of Public Health assured the Ministry of Commerce that it would take the strongest stand possible up to the last minute in order to increase Thailand's bargaining power but that it would not be unrea-sonable if time ran out, since it wanted to avoid trade retaliation. With this assurance, the Ministry of Commerce seemed much more at ease with the MOPH and worked together with it until the GATT ruling. The coopera-tion was so successful that the permanent secretary of the Ministry of Commerce suggested that it was an opportune time to reorient Thailand's tobacco control policy in response to the government's embarrassment over the forced opening of the Thai market. With that encouragement, the MOPH proposed to the cabinet a Tobacco Product Control bill and the establishment of the Tobacco Consumption Control Office (TCCO). Both were approved.

Interestingly, proof of health damage from tobacco did not come from Thai research. Thailand has not systematically carried out research on tobacco control issues, and studies from other countries and WHO recom-mendations were used in lobbying for policy and legislation. For example, data from the U.S. Environmental Protection Agency, as well as the U.S. Surgeon General's report (USDHHS 1986), were used to lobby for the law banning smoking in public places. In 1988 Richard Peto recommended that

Thailand undertake several tobacco-related research studies for tobacco control. When Peto returned to Thailand in 2001 to receive the prestigious Prince Mahidol Award for his contributions to public health, the author apologized to him for not carrying out the research he had recommended. Peto replied, "Never mind, you got the job done. Two million Thais have quit smoking and the smoking rate is down. That's what matters." In his press briefing, Peto said, "Thailand is really unique among developing countries. It has managed to get a significant reduction in men who smoke. A quarter of middle-aged men in Thailand have stopped smoking, which is quite different from China and India, where there has been little change in smoking patterns" (*Bangkok Post* 2001).

Thailand has been able to move tobacco control forward using credible evidence from research in other countries, but its success has come in large part because of the role of organizations such as Mahidol University and the efforts of credible spokespersons. Research is still needed, but if action is delayed by demands for country-specific proof, many countries may never be able to make speedy progress in tobacco control. It is not uncommon for some politicians to request evidence from research as a pretext to block or delay tobacco control measures.

The Sometimes Fine Art of Raising Tobacco Taxes

Increasing the tobacco tax was an idea that had first been considered in 1988 as part of the package of tobacco control measures proposed by the MOPH to the cabinet, but it never moved forward. In 1989, during the trade negotiations with the United States, the TASCP and the NCCTU proposed a tax increase, but that too went nowhere because the government did not want to anger the U.S. Trade Office. The minister of public health said that he did not wish to propose a tax, arguing that it was a matter for the minister of finance. In turn, the minister of finance claimed that he did not need additional revenues at the time. The impasse was typical of Thai politicians, who hate to lose popularity, especially among the many voters who smoke. (In fact, surveys in country after country find that most people, including a majority of smokers, support increases in tobacco taxes; see, for example, Environics Research Group 2001.)

In 1993 Supakorn Buasai of the Health Systems Research Institute (HSRI), Neil Collishaw of the WHO tobacco control program, and the author, as secretary to the NCCTU, urged the minister of public health, Arthit Ourairat, to raise the excise tax on cigarettes (Buasai 1993; Collishaw 1993). On the advice of David Sweanor of Canada's Non-Smokers' Rights Association, the group decided to argue in favor of taxation as a means of preventing children from smoking. "You just tell them how many children will be prevented [from smoking] and walk away," said

Sweanor. No request for money for tobacco control was made, so no accusations of self-interest could be claimed.

Judith Mackay, a recognized authority in Asian tobacco control who was in town at the time, joined in at a dinner with Minister Ourairat to lobby for the tax increase. The argument was put forth that since Thailand had a government-owned tobacco monopoly, there were only two policy options for generating tobacco revenues. The first was to let the tax stay low and sell more cigarettes. The second was to increase the tax, which would decrease cigarette sales and the number of people who smoked while increasing government revenue—a win-win situation. To avoid public criticism, the MOPH would propose the tax increase, allowing the Ministry of Finance to appear to play a neutral role. To get the tax approved, however, there had to be at least tacit approval by the minister of finance, since he was from the Democrat Party, while Ourairat was from the Seritham Party.

During the lobbying of the cabinet members, Paibul Suriyawongpaisal, a faculty member at Ramathibodi Hospital, conducted a public opinion poll to highlight the level of support for a tobacco tax increase (Suriyawongpaisal 1993). Of the 1,000 Bangkok residents polled, 70 percent, including 60 percent of the smokers, favored the tax increase. These results were released to the press a few days before the cabinet meeting. The TTM strongly opposed the tax, arguing that the country would lose money and that the tax would worsen the already bad smuggling problem. Despite the great pressure on Ourairat to give up the tax increase plan, he eventually won. He emerged from the cabinet meeting saying, "Well, you have the tax increase. It was either that or finding a new public health minister."

This first tax increase in 1993 was from 55 to 60 percent, with a provision to adjust the tax for inflation. In 1994, according to the Excise Department (Ministry of Finance 2001), revenue from cigarette excise taxes jumped from 15 billion baht (US$0.576 billion) to 20 billion baht (US$0.769 billion). Since then, the tax has been increased six times and currently stands at 75 percent of the retail price.

Politicians in many countries are reluctant to take tobacco control measures, fearing harm to the economy. But their fears usually turn out not to fit the facts. Higher taxes raise revenues, and declines in sales of tobacco products may create many more new jobs in industries to which people switch their consumption than are lost in the tobacco industry as a result of lower sales. The World Bank regards tobacco control as a good investment. *World Development Report 1993* noted, "Tax policies on tobacco and alcohol have reduced consumption, especially by discouraging use by young adults before they become addicted" (p. 87), and a 1999 report on tobacco control stated, "For governments intent on improving health within the framework of sound economic policies, action to control tobacco represents an unusually attractive choice" (p. x). Thailand's experience demonstrates that increased tobacco taxation is good for both public health and the economy. The Thai government has gained over 40 billion baht (US$1 billion) in additional revenues through cigarette tax increases, while smoking prevalence fell from 26.3 percent in 1992 to 20.5 percent in 1999 (National Statistics Office 1999; Ministry of Finance 2001).

Toward a Dedicated Tax for Health Promotion

A decade after its formation, the TASCP changed its name to Action on Smoking and Health (ASH) and became independent of the Folk Doctors Foundation. The organization had gained credibility largely because of its role in the Thai–U.S. trade dispute and the tobacco excise tax struggle. That credibility helped the group continue its advocacy for tobacco control when, in 1996, the Ministry of Finance organized a workshop on fiscal policy for social development as part of the government's decentralization policy. Out of that workshop emerged the idea of using tax revenues for a health insurance scheme and for health promotion.

Coincidentally, at the same time the Health Systems Research Institute held a conference in Bangkok on organizational structures for health promotion in developing countries. Rhonda Galbally, chief executive officer of the Victorian Health Promotion Foundation (VicHealth), Australia, was one of the keynote speakers. VicHealth is a statutory autonomous organization that has been funded by a dedicated tobacco tax since 1987. The WHO had recommended that member countries adopt the VicHealth model for health promotion (Galbally 1997). Supakorn Buasai, deputy director of the HSRI, and the author took advantage of Galbally's presence and, after the conference, accompanied her to meet with the minister of finance, Dr. Surakiat Steinthai, who seemed open to the idea of investing in health promotion. After that meeting, at the request of the minister, a small Thai delegation went to Australia and New Zealand to examine how VicHealth used a dedicated tax to promote health.

The delegation worked on proposed legislation that would set up a Health Promotion Office as an autonomous agency within the Prime Minister's Office. It recommended a dedicated tax of 2.5 to 3 percent of the tobacco tax, or about 700 million baht (US$27 million) per year, to fund the office. The sum would be equivalent to about 1 percent of the MOPH's yearly budget. The permanent secretary of the Ministry of Finance opposed the idea of a dedicated tax, but the final decision was to let the cabinet determine the source of the funds.

Progress on this matter halted in July 1997, when the Asian financial crisis hit Thailand. Work on the health promotion bill did not resurface until 1999. During this period, Dr. Phisit Leeartham, a banker who was invited by the Democrat Party to be deputy minister of finance during the economic crisis, was admitted to Ramathibodi Hospital as a patient. When the author, in his capacity as dean of the university hospital, visited Leeartham, the deputy minister promised to help move the health promotion bill forward.

Two months later, the MOPH called a meeting to consider a bill, drafted by the Excise Department, to reduce alcohol and tobacco consumption. A proposal was made to fund the program with a 2 percent dedicated tax on alcohol and tobacco. This came as a big surprise in light of previous resistance to a dedicated tax. The proposed Health Promotion Office bill had a good structure but no funding source; the new bill from the Excise Department had specific funding provisions but few administrative details (HSRI 1997).

After this meeting, Leeartham (who gave the green light for the dedicated tax) suggested that health promotion be added throughout the alcohol and tobacco bill and the name changed to "A Bill to Set up a Fund for a Campaign to Reduce Alcohol and Tobacco Consumption and for Health Promotion." He also suggested that the Health Promotion Office bill and the new bill to fund the campaign not be combined, since that would be too time consuming (a concern, as the government's popularity was waning). Rather, he proposed that the two bills be submitted to the cabinet at the same time. The idea was to set up a Health Promotion Office and start carrying out health promotion activities with an initial budget while waiting for the funding bill to make its way through Parliament.

The cabinet spent over two hours debating whether the Health Promotion Office should be supervised by the minister of health or should be an autonomous organization under the Prime Minister's Office. Prime Minister Leekpai finally agreed to the latter. The minister of public health, who represented a different political party, was unhappy with this decision, and the MOPH had a limited role during the rest of the bill's journey into law.

In October 1999 the cabinet approved both bills and sent them to be reviewed by the Council of State. (It should be noted that the prime minister showed a keen interest in solving alcohol-related problems. His support of the lobby made things easier, since the Democrat Party controlled the cabinet as well as the House of Representatives.) The bill for the Health Promotion Office was approved first, and 152 million baht (about US$3.5 million) was allocated for the office's first year of operation. Meanwhile, a lobby began in favor of naming Athasit Vejjajiva, a politically influential figure, as the office's first chairperson. The aim was to strengthen the political status of the bill by appointing someone who was politically astute and trustworthy.

Clearing the alcohol and tobacco use reduction and health promotion bill through the Council of State was more difficult because of the provision for the dedicated tax. To help push it along, it was moved to a different committee of the council, and its name was changed to "A Bill to Set up Funding for Health Promotion." Eventually, it was steered through three readings in the Lower House and finally to passage in the last session of the Parliament. Unfortunately, the bill did not get through the Senate in the last two days of the parliamentary session. This meant that it would have to be approved by the newly elected government before being taken up again in the Senate. Luckily the new government's health policy included universal health coverage, and it was easily convinced that health promotion fit well into its agenda. The government endorsed the bill's introduction in the Senate—one among only 27 of the 45 bills remaining from the previous government that were reintroduced.

But the challenges did not end there. Under the new constitution, the Senate was elected, not appointed, making it more difficult to steer the bill through. In what seemed to be an effort to increase their own popularity and visibility, some senators seemed delighted to highlight objections to the bill, claiming that it was unnecessary, or that it set a bad precedent, or that there should not be an autonomous organization. Interestingly, those who objected the most were doctors who were former bureaucrats in the MOPH.

The bill finally passed in the Senate on September 26, 2001. It was signed by the king on October 27 and published in the *Royal Gazette* in early November, thus becoming law. The Health Promotion Office was already in operation, and the passage of the funding bill secured its future. The Senate, however, specified in a footnote to the bill that a dedicated tax would be allowed this time only and that future governments should not propose a law of this kind again. Much concern was expressed about the appropriate use of the relatively high budget of the Health Promotion Office (14 billion baht, or US$35 million per year, compared with 12 million baht, or US$300,000 per year, for the MOPH's Tobacco Consumption Control Office). Under Vejjajiva's chairmanship of the board of the Thai Health Promotion Office, tobacco control efforts have grown dramatically from the initial allocation of 60,000 baht (US$2,255) for a project in 1986 to its current budget and a range of activities that includes health promotion as well as reduction of tobacco and alcohol use.

Continuing Opposition from the Tobacco Companies

Let it not be thought that the international tobacco industry was inattentive or inactive in blocking, delaying, or seeking to weaken tobacco policy in Thailand. The industry's successful petition to the U.S. administration to use Section 301 against Thailand clearly showed its intentions. Its lobbying to repeal the sports sponsorship ban early on demonstrated its understanding of the tools that could be used to change the marketing environment quickly.

One of the early challenges following the GATT decision was the issue of sports sponsorship. The tobacco industry worked closely with sports associations, sportswriters, and even government sports officials to lobby the government to repeal the advertising ban and allow sports sponsorship. One association after another explicitly or tacitly succumbed to the industry, and the press reported growing support for tobacco sports sponsorship.

The TASCP worked closely with Chitanondh in opposing this trend. Several strategies were pursued: launching a counterattack in the media by having an ex-smoker sportswriter voice support for the sponsorship ban; producing a report explaining why cigarette companies should not sponsor sports and referring to the Olympic Charter banning cigarette sponsorship; and proposing a sports fund funded by a tobacco tax like the one in Australia. In 1991 Privy Council Member Prem Tinsulanonda (the former prime minister whose cabinet had issued the ministerial regulation banning tobacco advertising and sponsorship) made a strong statement that sports sponsorship by tobacco companies was inappropriate, and the matter was laid to rest.

This struggle is just one illustration of how the tobacco industry operates. In fact, recently released tobacco industry documents show that the industry views tobacco control advocates as competitors for their market (Philip Morris 1994).

Even after the advertising ban, tobacco companies found ways to promote their products. Philip Morris soon announced a program of art sponsorship in Southeast Asia, and it now holds an annual Association of Southeast Asian Nations (ASEAN) arts contest in a different ASEAN country each year. The international tobacco companies have also taken full advantage of the ASEAN Free Trade Agreement (AFTA) by moving their production facilities to ASEAN countries so that their products are subject to lower tariffs and are much more competitive with local brands (Vateesatokit, Hughes, and Ritthphakdee 2000). Now the most popular foreign brand, L&M, is cheaper than the most popular Thai brand, Krong Thip.

The AFTA tariff reduction has resulted in a marked increase in foreign brands' market share since 1999. In 2001 foreign brands accounted for 15 percent of the legal market and an unknown (but likely very high) portion of the illegal market. Internal tobacco industry documents strongly suggest that illegal sales and price fixing have been used in Thailand to systematically build brand popularity (*Economist* 2001). The industry was also keen to obtain some form of joint venture with the TTM (Hammond 1999).

The international tobacco companies have continued to use indirect advertising and point-of-sale promotions, in violation of Thai law (ASH Thailand n.d.). To gain favor, they use corporate donations to fund high-profile projects and charitable organizations such as population and family planning associations, as well as the Bangkok Metropolitan Administration. They also introduced the "18-plus" project, putting up stickers in retail shops reminding consumers that selling cigarettes to people under age 18 is illegal. While this may seem like a step toward tobacco control, ASH has found that this project actually stimulates interest in smoking by young people.

In comparison with the international companies, the TTM has seemed rather benign, but it has slowly adopted some of the strategies of the internationals. It began using corporate image advertising and hired a private company to do market research aimed at modernizing its marketing approach. It also strongly opposed the introduction on Thai cigarette packaging of pictorial health warnings like those used in Canada.

The Role of the Nongovernmental Sector

When the TASCP was first formed, it had only two part-time staff: Bung-On Ritthphakdee and the author. Up to 1992, most efforts concentrated on the U.S.–Thai trade struggle and the two resulting Thai laws, but by 1994 there was a marked increase in activity. Several programs were operating by that time, ranging from tobacco industry surveillance to promoting smoke-free homes and schools. The number of programs has grown, and their scope has greatly expanded to include both regional and international cooperation and collaboration on many aspects of tobacco control. Currently, the TASCP's successor, ASH, has 10 full-time staff and derives funding from the MOPH, the WHO, corporate and private donations, and fund-raising activities.

Recently, ASH has added tobacco control research to its list of activities. In 1998 it received funding from the HSRI to be the tobacco information clearinghouse for Thailand and to develop and contract research proposals with university researchers on topics such as the social and economic causes of cigarette smoking, the role of health professionals in tobacco control, and women and tobacco. ASH has developed a strong working relationship with the National Office of Statistics and with other research institutes that gather useful policy-driven data on tobacco control.

In 2000 the Rockefeller Foundation funded ASH as the center for the Southeast Asia Tobacco Control Alliance. Several previous attempts by ASH to form a network or coalition of health groups against tobacco had been unsuccessful, partly because of lack of funding support, so this new support was a huge boost. The main objective of the alliance is to train health professionals in research for tobacco control in the region, with assistance from the Institute for Global Tobacco Control, Johns Hopkins University in Baltimore, and the University of Illinois, Chicago. Potential topics for future research include smuggling; counteradvertising; international trade laws and their impact on tobacco consumption, global trade, and privatization; and smoking and drug abuse. Such research provides an important mechanism for recruiting health professionals and other academics to carry out tobacco control research, policy development, and program implementation.

The activities of ASH/TASCP represent the core of NGO actions in Thailand, but the government counterpart, the Tobacco Consumption Control Office (TCCO) of the MOPH, has also been important. This office was set up in 1991 to serve as secretariat to the NCCTU. Early on, the TASCP and the TCCO worked hand in hand, complementing each other in carrying forward tobacco control programs. The TASCP worked on advocacy and campaign activities, while the TCCO focused on law enforcement and policy formation. It was unfortunate that this complementary, productive relationship was later disrupted because of the frequent changes in government and some conflict as to approaches.

Ten years after the legal entry of international tobacco companies into the Thai market, the close consultation on tobacco control policy among the Ministries of Public Health, Finance, and Commerce no longer exists. The MOPH still has a strong policy on tobacco control, but it has not taken a tough stand with international companies on ingredient disclosure. In response to opposition from the tobacco companies, it has also delayed its proposal to revise the health warning to a pictorial format, as proposed by ASH.

Meanwhile, the Ministry of Commerce wants the MOPH to consult it on any future regulations affecting cigarette sales, to avoid friction with the U.S. Trade Office. And the Ministry of Finance quietly proceeded with the TTM's privatization plan to fulfill its obligation to the International Monetary Fund (IMF) to privatize state enterprises—a condition of the financial assistance package provided to Thailand during the 1997 economic crisis. The ministry backtracked at the last minute under pressure from tobacco control advocates, who oppose privatization of cigarette manufacturers because they believe it is likely to give multinational companies greater leverage and a stronger base from which to lobby against and undermine tobacco control.

Despite all this, the three ministries have been careful to appear supportive of tobacco control policy in light of the strong antismoking sentiment of the Thai public.

Spreading the Message: Thai Women Do Not Smoke

Thailand has long felt that preventing women from smoking is a neglected area in tobacco control programs and research worldwide. The Kobe Declaration of the 1999 WHO International Conference on Tobacco or Health states, "It is urgent that we find comprehensive solutions to the danger of tobacco use and address the epidemic among women and girls" (Ernster and others 2000).

Smoking among Thai women is not widely accepted culturally, and fewer than 5 percent of them smoke. But over the years there have been efforts by the tobacco industry to capture the female market. Before the opening of the Thai tobacco market to foreign cigarettes, the TTM tried marketing a cigarette specifically to females—fortunately, without success. But there was concern that when the market did open, the targeted advertising and marketing of international companies would succeed in attracting women to smoke. That certainly was the experience in Japan and Taiwan (China), where the number of women smoking increased dramatically after the markets opened (Chaloupka and Laixuthai 1996).

Following the GATT decision, Greg Connolly suggested lobbying the Thai government to restrict the introduction of brands targeting women, citing the low smoking rate among Thai females. These efforts failed because the head of the Thai negotiating team, Bajr Israsena, did not want any further trouble with the U.S. Trade Office and thought that the ban would be contrary to GATT provisions. As a result, Virginia Slims, a brand of cigarettes marketed to women, was soon introduced in Thailand.

Faced with the import of cigarettes targeted at women, the TASCP in 1994 set up the Thai Women Do Not Smoke Project, with the objective of preserving the nonsmoking norm among Thai women. The TASCP used research by Dr. Varanut Wangsuphachart and others (1995) showing that smoking was common only among women in certain occupations (47 percent of massage parlor workers, 10 percent of airline hostesses, and less than 10 percent of all other groups). The project was supported by Miss Thailand and a number of young movie and television stars, who acted as presenters for the program.

In 1996, five years after the opening of the market to foreign cigarettes, the TTM announced that it would begin marketing a brand of cigarette to women to compete with Virginia Slims. ASH mobilized influential Thai women to oppose this move. Women members of Parliament, celebrities, and writers all joined in the campaign. Kanjana Silap-acha, daughter of the prime minister at the time, Banharn Silap-acha, lobbied her father to ask the minister of finance to request the TTM to cancel introduction of the new brand. All these efforts resulted in the TTM's dropping its plans to introduce "women's" cigarettes.

Mackay (1999), using a mathematical model that extrapolates smoking trends, and incorporating data from other countries as well, has predicted that smoking by women could rise to about 15 percent in Thailand over the next 25 years, while smoking by men could drop to about 25 percent. Several recent research projects on smoking by girls and women seem to support this projection. They show increasing smoking rates by girls in secondary school, with uptake mostly of foreign brands of cigarettes. It is hoped that this trend can be prevented in Thailand, since social pressure against women's smoking is still very strong and the advertising ban prevents the tobacco industry from targeting females.

Successes and Challenges

Thailand's tobacco control efforts, by the government and by NGOs, have achieved much. For example,

- Currently Thailand has a strong, comprehensive tobacco control policy.
- At a meeting convened by the National Committee for the Control of Tobacco Use on September 20, 2001, two committees were set up to evaluate the Tobacco Product Control Act and the Nonsmokers' Health Protection Act of 1992 after 10 years of existence. These committees will consider upgrading the laws to close loopholes and to strengthen law enforcement processes.
- The regular tax increase policy is on course.
- The current health warnings, which occupy the upper third of the two largest areas of cigarette packages and which have been in use for four years, will be revised to have a pictorial format, as championed by Garfield Mahood in Canada.
- The government has indefinitely halted privatization of the TTM. It had seemed impossible to stop privatization because it was part of the IMF bailout package following the 1997 economic crisis. Work continued, however, even when the situation seemed hopeless, and eventually public health considerations prevailed.
- Thailand will continue to take a very strong position on international issues such as trade, duty-free sales, smuggling, and transboundary advertising and promotion.
- Tobacco control is and will be the main project for the new Thai Health Promotion Foundation.
- The Thai Women Do Not Smoke project is being funded by the Thai Health Promotion Foundation.

But success has not been won on every front. More work remains to be done.

Ingredient Disclosure

In 1989, at the public hearings in Washington, D.C., on the Section 301 case, David Sweanor of Canada's Non-Smokers' Rights Association stated that he did not think Thailand could win its trade case. He recommended trying to pass a law with a provision on ingredient disclosure, which would deter American manufacturers from exporting to Thailand, and he gave the Thai representatives a copy of the Canadian Tobacco Products Control Act of 1988. This document was used as a basis for Thailand's Tobacco Product Control Bill, which closely followed the Canadian law.

In 1990 the cabinet approved the law, including, in Article 11, the provision on ingredient disclosure. But in 1992, when the bill was presented to Parliament for the second reading, the international tobacco industry lobbied extensively for deletion of both Article 4 (a provision barring sales to minors under age 18) and Article 11. It was clear that the real intention was to get Article 11 deleted, since worldwide evidence showed that laws barring sales to minors are nearly impossible to enforce.

The lobby was so intense that Deputy Minister Vejjajiva informed the author that saving Article 11 appeared unlikely. Sensing the author's despair, Vejjajiva called General Suchinda Kraprayoon, who held the real power, having been the strongman in the 1991 coup in Thailand and having directed the formation of the interim administration and legislature. He gave the green light for the bill to sail through with Article 11 intact, which empowered the minister of public health to issue a ministerial regulation regarding ingredient disclosure.

Despite the passage of the law, the ministers of health in 1992 and 1993 took no action on drafting a regulation. Finally, in 1995, Minister Ourairat pushed it through in the last cabinet meeting of his government for the year. When the Council of State considered the regulation, the international tobacco companies tried to have a say but were turned down. Even then, it took two more years before the regulation was signed into law by Minister of Public Health Montree Pongpanich. The tobacco companies were given six months from the time of signing to comply with the regulation.

Still, the challenge did not end. When the government changed, the officials of the new MOPH refused to reveal to the public the list of ingredients submitted by the tobacco industry, on the grounds that doing so would interfere with the ability of the Ministry of Commerce to deal with international trade issues. The intensity of the tobacco industry's lobbying against this type of law in Thailand and the injunctive action against a similar regulation in the U.S. state of Massachusetts led to widespread suspicion of intervention by the international tobacco industry.

So, after all that, the attempt to use a disclosure regulation to prevent more harmful cigarettes from entering the market and to keep out foreign cigarettes did not succeed. At present, the law is useless, but not forgotten. Perhaps another opportunity will come.

Other Challenges

There are two other areas in which success has not been achieved: removing cigarettes from the duty-free list, and removing them from the AFTA free trade zone. Cigarettes remain duty-free because government officials fear that a change would affect Thailand's profitable tourist industry. Thailand was unable to persuade other ASEAN countries to drop cigarettes from the AFTA list of free trade items. It is hoped that the Framework Convention on Tobacco Control will assist countries like Thailand to take the strongest stand possible regarding international trade and other issues and to do so effectively (Framework Convention Alliance 2001).

Lessons Learned

Lessons can be drawn from both the successes and the frustrations of the struggle for tobacco control. Some of these are specific to the Thai context, but many are more widely applicable.

Working with Legislators and Regulators

- Regulators often have very specific opinions on the proposals before them, and even with the best evidence, they are not always prepared to change their minds (Pertschuk 2001). The Thai experience shows that when key people oppose proposals and support other interests, it is important to wait until more favorable views surface, perhaps after a change of leadership, and to seize favorable opportunities when they arise. Between 1989 and 2001, Thailand had 9 governments and 11 ministers of health, and progress on tobacco control often stalled. At least one minister of health during this time was referred to in tobacco industry documents as "our friend in MOPH" (Le Gresley n.d.). Other ministers, however, have been highly supportive of tobacco control.
- Those with opposing views and interests are well aware that tobacco control advocates will guard and protect hard-earned gains. By maintaining dialogue with key individuals and agencies, the tobacco control lobby was able to gain a clearer idea of how to proceed.
- When lobbying for tax increases and for legislation, it could be a good strategy to make clear to policymakers that the objective is to prevent children from smoking and becoming addicted to nicotine.

Most people support this goal unequivocally, even if they waver with respect to actions aimed at persuading adult smokers to quit.

- The effort to pass tobacco control legislation wherever possible should be sustained, since governments come and go but repealing or revising already-enacted legislation is time consuming and costly.

Working with Politicians

- Ultimate goals have to be balanced against reasonable expectations. In Thailand the ultimate goal was to prevent the government from opening the tobacco market to imports, but the lobbying group settled on passing the Tobacco Product Control Bill and setting up the Tobacco Consumption Control Office. Politicians recognized that they had a responsibility to the public to do something to decrease the health risks of smoking. Using a moral argument was particularly useful in Thailand's government system.

- In Thailand there appears to be a difference between the "technocrat turned politician" and the "career politician." Most of the achievements in tobacco control policy and legislation in Thailand resulted from working with technocrats who seemed to decide policy on the basis of objectivity and the value of the issue itself. Most career politicians (perhaps with the exceptions of Chuan Leekpai and Surin Pitsuwan) seemed to be more concerned with balancing vested interests against their own popularity, and they would often avoid making decisions on controversial issues. By contrast, Athasit Vejjajiva, a technocrat minister, was a key figure in moving the two tobacco control bills forward through the cabinet and eventually to Parliament, and Arthit Ourairat, a technocrat turned politician, supported the tax for health policy in 1993. Phisit Leeartham, another technocrat, was the central strategist in moving the Health Promotion Bill, with the dedicated tax, which may go down in Thai history as the only one of its kind. It is not clear whether these milestones would have been achieved by relying on career politicians only.

- It is important to be direct, clear, and ready with realistic proposals to offer politicians. At times, seemingly controversial political personalities, shunned by others, were found to be most supportive.

- In order to ensure that antitobacco policies are adopted, it may help to allow bureaucrats and politicians to claim credit for new initiatives.

- Personal connections are often invaluable in helping to secure desired policy outcomes.

- A politician's support should never be taken for granted. Showing appreciation, along with hard work and good evidence, is key to moving tobacco control onto the agenda of politicians.

The Importance of Organizational Understanding and Collaboration

- It is essential to have a lead organization to push for tobacco control in both the nongovernmental and governmental sectors. Ideally, collaboration between the two sectors should enhance each other's work.
- Networking and coalition building, both domestically and internationally, are crucial to increasing the lobbying power of tobacco control advocates.

The Importance of Well-Prepared Evidence and Good Cultural Understanding

- Health education is important but is insufficient by itself for effective tobacco control.
- Policy-relevant research is very important in mobilizing public opinion and lobbying for government action.
- Gaining Ministry of Finance cooperation in using taxation as a control measure was easier once the evidence about the health care costs of smoking and the potential increase in revenues was presented.
- Nationalism and cultural values can sometimes be successfully employed to counter tobacco promotion by international tobacco companies.
- Tobacco control advocates should seize opportunities to make timely counterclaims to arguments by pro-tobacco lobbyists.

Appendix: Chronological Summary of Tobacco Control Efforts in Thailand

World War II–1990: The Thai government owns the tobacco monopoly and has a closed market. The smoking rate is very high for males, with average annual per capita consumption of about 1,000 cigarettes.

1970s: The Thai Medical Association initiates tobacco control by printing health warnings, banning smoking in cinemas and on buses, and conducting a national survey of smoking prevalence.

1976–86: Sporadic smoking control activities are carried out by government agencies and nongovernmental organizations.

1986: The Thai Anti-Smoking Campaign Project (TASCP) is formed to serve as a focal point and pressure group in lobbying for tobacco control policy.

1989: The U.S. Trade Representative, using Section 301 of the U.S. Trade Act, brings the issue of tobacco control to national and international attention, culminating in the GATT adjudication, the eventual market opening, and the Thai government's approval of the Tobacco Product Control Bill.

1992: The National Legislative Assembly enacts the Tobacco Product Control Bill and the Nonsmokers' Health Protection Bill despite heavy lobbying by the tobacco industry.

1993: Health advocates successfully lobby for the tax for health policy; the Thai government gains huge revenue increases, and per capita consumption of cigarettes is curbed.

1994: The TASCP organizes the Thai Women Do Not Smoke Project to discourage Thai women from taking up smoking.

1996: The TASCP, renamed Action on Smoking and Health (ASH), successfully lobbies the Thai government to call off the Thai Tobacco Monopoly's plan to market a cigarette brand targeted to women.

1998: The ingredient disclosure regulation of the Tobacco Product Control Act is passed into law, but the Ministry of Public Health is unwilling to reveal the ingredient list to the public, thus defeating any potential benefit.

2001: The Health Promotion Bill, funded by a dedicated alcohol and tobacco tax, is finally enacted in September, after five years of lobbying.

2002: Plans for privatization of the Thai Tobacco Monopoly are put on "indefinite hold," after seeming to be unstoppable.

References

ASH (Action on Smoking and Health) Thailand. n.d. "Point of Sale Advertising for Cigarettes in Thailand." Available at <http://www.ashthailand.or.th/en/informationcenter_en.php?act=list_category>; accessed Jan. 13, 2003.

Bangkok Post. 2001. "AFP: Thai Anti-Smoking Drive Wins Praise." Feb. 2, p. 5.

Buasai, S. 1993. "The Increase of the Excise Tax." Paper submitted for consideration by the Thai cabinet, Dec. 7.

Chaloupka, F. J., and A. Laixuthai. 1996. "U.S. Trade Policy and Cigarette Smoking in Asia." Working Paper 5543. National Bureau of Economic Research, Cambridge, Mass. Available at <http://papers.nber.org/papers/w5543>.

Chantornvong, S., and D. McCargo. 2001. "Political Economy of Tobacco Control in Thailand." *Tobacco Control* 10 (1): 48–54. Available at <http://tc.bmjjournals.com/cgi/content/full/10/1/48>.

Chen, T. L., and W. M. Elaimy. 1994. "APACT: Development and Challenges in the Face of Adversity." *Proceedings of the Third Asia-Pacific Conference on Tobacco or Health, June 1993, Omiya, Japan,* 319–24. Tokyo: Asia-Pacific Association for the Control of Tobacco.

Chitanondh, H. 2001. "Defeat in Trade, Victory in Health." Thailand Health Promotion Institute, Bangkok.

Collishaw, N. 1993. "Potential Health Benefits of a 10% Increase in the Real Price of Tobacco through Taxation in Thailand." Press release. Health Systems Research Institute, Ministry of Public Health, Bangkok.

Deerasamee, S., and others, ed. 1999. *Cancer in Thailand.* Vol. 2: *1992–1994.* IARC Technical Report 34. Lyon: International Agency for Research on Cancer.

Economist. 2001. "The Price Is Not Quite Right: Cigarette Companies Have Been Accused of All Sorts of Wrongdoing. Is It Time to Add Price-Fixing to the List?" July 5.

Ekplakorn, W., W. Wongkraisrithong, and S. Tangchareonsin. 1991. "Epidemiology of Smoking-Related Diseases in Thailand." Epidemiology Division, Office of the Permanent Secretary, Ministry of Public Health, Bangkok.

Environics Research Group. 2001. "Public Support for International Efforts to Control Tobacco. A Survey in Five Countries." Toronto.

Ernster, V., and others. 2000. "Women and Tobacco: Moving from Policy to Action." *Bulletin of the World Health Organization* 78 (7): 891–901.

Framework Convention Alliance. 2001. "Briefing Paper: Trade Issues and the Recommended Text." Bangkok. Available at <http://www.fctc.org/INB3brief_trade.pdf>; cited Oct. 13, 2001.

Frankel, G. 1996. "Big Tobacco's Global Reach: Thailand Resists US Brand Assault; Stiff Laws Inspire Other Asians to Curb Smoking." *Washington Post,* Nov. 18, p. A1.

Galbally, R. 1997. "The Victorian Health Foundation." Paper presented at the Regional Workshop on Organizational and Funding Infrastructure, November 1997, Bangkok. Health Systems Research Institute, Ministry of Public Health, and WHO Regional Office, Bangkok.

GATT (General Agreement on Tariffs and Trade). 1990. "Decision: Thailand Restrictions on Importation of and Internal Taxes on Cigarettes," bisd 37S/200. World Trade Organization, Geneva.

Hammond, R. 1999. "Big Tobacco's Overseas Expansion: Focus on Thailand." Case study. San Francisco Tobacco Free Project, San Francisco, Calif.

HSRI (Health Systems Research Institute). 1997. "Health Promotion Fund." Draft proposal. Bangkok.

Le Gresley, E. n.d. Personal communication.

Mackay, J. 1999. "Tobacco Control Now and in the Future." Paper presented at the Together Against Tobacco Meeting, INGCAT International NGO Mobilization Meeting, May 1999, Geneva. International Nongovernmental Coalition Against Tobacco, Paris.

Ministry of Finance, Excise Department. 1994. *Annual Report: Cigarette Sales and Tax Revenue 1993.* Bangkok.

———. 1999. *Production Report of the Thai Tobacco Monopoly.* Bangkok.

———. 2001. *Cigarette Sales and Tax Revenue 1993–2001.* Bangkok.

Muscat, R. J. 1992. *The Fifth Tiger: A Study of Thai Development Policy.* New York: United Nations University Press.

National Statistics Office. 1999. *National Health and Welfare Survey.* Bangkok.

Pertschuk, M. 2001. "The Power of Science and Truth: Countering Paid Liars' Efforts to Influence Tobacco Policy." *Tobacco Control* 10 (3): 225–26. Available at <http://tc.bmjjournals.com/cgi/content/full/10/3/225>.

Philip Morris. 1994. "The Increase of Consumption Restrictions Worldwide." Global Situation Analysis Report. New York. Bates no. 2045655906/5934; available at <http://www.pmdocs.com/getallimg.asp?DOCID=2045655906/5934>; cited March 1, 2002.

Supawongse, C., ed. 1999. *Evolution of Tobacco Consumption Control in Thailand.* Bangkok: Department of Health, Ministry of Public Health.

Suriyawongpaisal, P. 1993. "Bangkok Residents Support Cigarette Tax." Press release. Thai Anti-Smoking Campaign Project, Bangkok.

TASCP (Thai Anti-Smoking Campaign Project). 1986. "Proceedings of the Seminar 'Cigarettes: A Silent Danger Undermining Society,' November 1986, Bangkok." Bangkok.

———. 1988. "One Million Children Will Eventually Die from Smoking." Press release. Bangkok.

Tobacco Merchants Association. 1988. "US Cigarette Export Market Penetration in Thailand: A Multimillion Dollar Opportunity for US Leaf Producers." Princeton, N.J.

USDHHS (U.S. Department of Health and Human Services). 1986. The Health Consequences of Involuntary Smoking: A Report of the Surgeon General. Publ. CDC 87-8398. Atlanta, Ga.

Vateesatokit, P. 1990a. "Resisting the Tobacco Industry in Asia." Paper presented at the 15th International Cancer Conference, August, 1990, Hamburg, Germany. International Union against Cancer.

———. 1990b. "Tobacco and Trade Sanctions: The Next Victim after Thailand." In Tobacco and Health 1990: The Global War. Proceedings of the Seventh Conference on Tobacco or Health, April 1990, Perth, Australia. Geneva: World Health Organization.

———. 1996. "Tobacco Control in Thailand." Siriraj Hospital Gazette 48 (suppl.): 119–52.

———. 1997. "Tobacco Control in Thailand." Mahidol Journal 4 (2): 73–84.

———. 2001. "Thai Tobacco Control: Development through Strategic Alliances." Development Bulletin 54 (April): 63–66.

Vateesatokit, P., B. Hughes, and B. Ritthphakdee. 2000. "Thailand: Winning Battles, but the War's Far from Over." Tobacco Control 9 (2): 122–27. Available at <http://tc.bmjjournals.com/cgi/content/full/9/2/122>.

Wangsuphachart, V., and others. 1995. "Cross Sectional Study of Cigarette Smoking among Women of Specific Occupations." Mahidol University Research Abstracts (Thailand).

World Bank. 1993. World Development Report 1993: Investing in Health. New York: Oxford University Press.

———. 1999. Curbing the Epidemic: Governments and the Economics of Tobacco Control. Development in Practice series. Washington, D.C.

Index

priorities and, 34; education of public and politicians and, 27, 32–33; funds to support, 22–23, 31–32; laws regarding, 29; lessons learned in, 31–36; maintaining strong alliance and, 34–35; politics and, 28–30, 32–34; role of nongovernmental organizations (NGOs) in, 6, 7, 20–28; standing up to opposition and, 35–36; working with media and, 32–34

Basis for the Implementation of a Tobacco Control Program (Goldfarb et al.), 48

BAT. *See* British American Tobacco

BATA (Bangladesh Anti-Tobacco Alliance), 17, 21, 31, 35; activities championed by, 27–28; efforts against BAT's Voyage of Discovery campaign and, 23–34, 26, 36; founding of, 22, 27; funding for, 22–23, 31–32; importance of, 24–28; mission of, 26–27; organizations in network of, 25–26. *See also individual organizations*; relationship with government and, 29–30; WHO's 2001 Tobacco Free World Award received by, 30

Beatty, Perrin, 83

Bhorer Kagoj, 29, 33

Biman, smoking prohibited on flights of, 29

Body Against Destructive Social Activities (BADSA) (Bangladesh), 25

Bornvornwattanuvongs, Jureerut, 157

Botha, P. W., 123

Bouchard, Benoit, 83

Brazil: development in, indicators of, 2, 4–5; economics of tobacco in, 39–40; export earnings from tobacco in, 39–40; government support for tobacco in, 40; illiteracy in, 4; life expectancy at birth in, 4; tobacco control in. *See* Brazil tobacco control; tobacco industry in, 54–55; tobacco production in, 39–40; tobacco product prices in, 45–46, 62–65; tobacco tax in, 66; tobacco use in, 4, 38–39, 45–46, 62, 65

Brazilian Cancer Society, 41

Brazilian Cigarettes: Analyses and Proposals to Reduce Consumption (Silva et al.), 47

Brazilian Medical Academy, 54

Brazilian Medical Association, 41

Brazilian Societies of Cardiology and Pediatrics, 54

Brazilian Tobacco Growers' Association (AFUBRA), 52, 55, 61–62

Brazil tobacco control, 11, 38–70; beginnings of, 40–42; business participation in, 42–43; "cascade" system for training and, 57–59; importance of partnerships and, 54; laws regarding, 6, 42, 45, 51–52, 55, 56–57; lessons learned in, 66–67; National Tobacco Control Program (NCTP) and, 42–52. *See also* NCTP; pictures to accompany warnings and, 57; public support and, 53–54; research projects and, 49–51; scope of Brazil's tobacco problem and, 38–40; taxation and, 66; tobacco industry opposition to, 54–55

British American Tobacco (BAT), 13, 16, 19, 157; advertising by, 21–22, 23, 29; attempts to resist regulation and, 17–18, 55; power of, 20; rock concerts sponsored by, 29; in South Africa, 122; Souza Cruz as Brazilian arm of, 55, 62; Voyage of Discovery campaign of, 21–22, 23–24, 26, 36

Brundtland, Gro Harlem, 149

BTC (Bangladesh Tobacco Company), 16

Buasai, Supakorn, 162, 164

Bush, George H. W., 159

CAB (Consumers' Association of Bangladesh), 25

Callard, Cynthia, 86

Canada: development in, indicators of, 2, 4–5; life expectancy at birth in, 2–3, 4; tobacco control in. *See* Canada tobacco control; tobacco industry in, 77–81, 93; tobacco production in, 72, 73–74; tobacco product prices in, 72, 74, 87–90, 91; tobacco tax in, 6, 71, 87–90, 94; tobacco use in, 3, 4, 71, 72–73, 87–90, 91, 92, 94

Canada tobacco control, 9, 71–96; advertising tug-of-war and, 77–81; budget for, 95; generation before,